CONQUER WORRY AND ANXIETY

THE SECRET TO MASTERING YOUR MIND

DANIEL G. AMEN, MD

TYNDALE
MOMENTUM®

The Tyndale nonfiction imprint

Visit Tyndale online at tyndale.com.

Visit Tyndale Momentum online at tyndalemomentum.com.

Visit Daniel G. Amen, MD, at http://www.amenclinics.com.

TYNDALE, *Tyndale Momentum*, and Tyndale's quill logo are registered trademarks of Tyndale House Publishers. The Tyndale Momentum logo is a trademark of Tyndale House Publishers. Tyndale Momentum is the nonfiction imprint of Tyndale House Publishers, Carol Stream, Illinois.

Conquer Worry and Anxiety: The Secret to Mastering Your Mind

Copyright © 2020 by Daniel G. Amen, MD. All rights reserved.

Adapted from *Feel Better Fast and Make It Last*, published in 2018 under ISBN 978-1-4964-2565-2, and *Stones of Remembrance*, published in 2017 under ISBN 978-1-4964-2667-3.

Cover illustration of mind mapping copyright © DrAfter123/Getty Images. All rights reserved.

Interior photographs, including brain scans and illustrations, provided by author and used with permission. All rights reserved.

Designed by Mark Anthony Lane II

Published in association with the literary agency of WordServe Literary Group, www.wordserveliterary.com.

Unless otherwise indicated, all Scripture quotations are taken from the *Holy Bible*, New Living Translation, copyright © 1996, 2004, 2015 by Tyndale House Foundation. Used by permission of Tyndale House Publishers, Carol Stream, Illinois 60188. All rights reserved.

Scripture quotations marked NIV are taken from the Holy Bible, *New International Version,*® *NIV.*® Copyright © 1973, 1978, 1984, 2011 by Biblica, Inc.® Used by permission. All rights reserved worldwide.

For information about special discounts for bulk purchases, please contact Tyndale House Publishers at csresponse@tyndale.com, or call 1-800-323-9400.

ISBN 978-1-4964-4659-6

Printed in the United States of America

26   25   24   23   22   21
7   6   5   4

MEDICAL DISCLAIMER

The information presented in this book is the result of years of practice experience and clinical research by the author. The information in this book, by necessity, is of a general nature and not a substitute for an evaluation or treatment by a competent medical specialist. If you believe you are in need of medical intervention, please see a medical practitioner as soon as possible. The stories in this book are true. The names and circumstances of some of the stories have been changed to protect the anonymity of patients.

Contents

Introduction

Don't worry about anything; instead, pray about everything. Tell God what you need, and thank him for all he has done. Then you will experience God's peace, which exceeds anything we can understand. His peace will guard your hearts and minds as you live in Christ Jesus.

PHILIPPIANS 4:6-7

IF YOU'RE LIKE ME, when you're feeling worried or anxious, you want to feel better now, fast, pronto! But many people, mental health professionals included, think therapy needs to be long, hard, and painful. They believe that if you start medication for anxiety or depression, you're making a lifelong commitment. Certainly, some people will need help longer than others, but in my experience, many people will feel better once they begin to engage in the right behaviors and strategies, which include knowing about and optimizing their brains.

Think about it: You know you can make yourself feel worse almost immediately by dwelling on the worst possible outcome of a situation, spending time with highly toxic people, or sabotaging each of your senses with dreadful sounds, smells, tastes, touches, or sights. You can just as easily make yourself feel better through simple choices like practicing gratitude, conquering negative thoughts, and using many other techniques that I will demonstrate throughout this book.

The truth is, we live in an impatient society. When people seek help for mental health issues, the most common number of therapy sessions they receive is one. Either they find benefit from getting their worries off their chests and learning simple strategies— or they conclude therapy won't be helpful for them. Even when they commit to ongoing therapy, the average number of sessions a patient attends is six or seven, regardless of the psychotherapist's theoretical orientation.[1]

Almost everyone wants to feel better fast, and research suggests it is possible. Studies since the 1980s have shown the value of single-session therapies (SSTs). In one study, a single session of hypnosis significantly decreased anxiety and depressive symptoms after coronary artery bypass surgery.[2] In another, Australian researchers found that 60 percent of children and teens with mental health issues showed improvement after 18 months from just one session of therapy.[3]

Helping people change their feelings and behaviors and optimize their lives has been my passion as a psychiatrist for the past four decades. Amen Clinics partnered with Professor BJ Fogg, director of the Persuasive Tech Lab at Stanford University, and his sister Linda Fogg-Phillips to help our patients with behavior change. They teach that only three things change behavior in the long run:

1. An epiphany
2. A change in the environment (what and who surrounds you)
3. Taking baby steps[4]

I once had an epiphany after reading a study by my friend Dr. Cyrus Raji[5] on what I call the dinosaur syndrome (as your weight goes up, the size and function of your brain go down—with a big body and a little brain, you're likely to become extinct). I then found the discipline to lose 25 pounds. But you don't have to wait for an epiphany to change your behavior. You don't need to experience daily panic attacks or get cancer in order to get serious about your health. When battling worry and anxiety, most people can change their environment (friends, workplace, church) or the people they surround themselves with, and all of us can make small changes that, over time, create amazing results.

High motivation helps you do hard things. But if your motivation is medium or even low, you can still change for the better. In fact, the Foggs encourage starting with baby steps, or what they call "Tiny Habits."[6] These are easy changes that will boost your sense of accomplishment and competence and, over time, evolve into bigger changes.

Here's one you can start right now that will make a huge and lasting change: Whenever you come to a decision point in your day, ask yourself, *Is the decision I'm about to make good for my brain or bad for it?*

If you consistently make decisions that serve your brain's health—and you'll learn more about how to do that in this book—you are well on your way to conquering worry and anxiety and living a happier, healthier life.

Daniel Amen, MD

CHAPTER 1

WHEN LIFE FEELS OUT OF CONTROL

Quick Calming Techniques

It is during our darkest moments that we must focus to see the light.

ATTRIBUTED TO ARISTOTLE

IT WAS 6:30 IN THE MORNING in the busy emergency room at the Walter Reed Army Medical Center in Washington, DC. I was just putting on my white lab coat as I walked through the doors to the unit. It was my third day as an intern, and the emergency room would be my home for the next month. Down the hall from me, a woman was screaming. Curious, I went to see what was going on.

Beth, a 40-year-old patient, was lying on a gurney with a swollen right leg. She was in obvious pain and screamed whenever anyone touched her leg. Bruce, a brand-new psychiatry intern like me, and Wendy, the internal medicine chief resident, were trying to start an IV in Beth's foot. She was anxious, scared, uncooperative, and hyperventilating. A blood clot in her calf was causing this tremendous swelling. The IV was necessary so Beth could be sent to the X-ray department for a scan that would show exactly where the clot was, allowing surgeons to operate and remove it. With each stick of the IV needle to her swollen foot, Beth's screams became louder. There was a lot of tension in the room.

"Wendy, can I try to start the IV?" I asked softly.

Exasperated, she handed me the IV set. I walked around the gurney to Beth's head, established eye contact with her, and gave her a gentle smile.

"Hi, Beth, I'm Dr. Amen. I need you to slow down your breathing. When you breathe too quickly, all of the blood vessels constrict, making it impossible for us to find a vein. Breathe with me." I slowed my own breathing.

"Do you mind if I help you relax?" I asked. "I know some tricks."

"Okay," Beth said nervously.

"Look at that spot on the ceiling," I said, pointing to a spot overhead. "I want you to focus on it and ignore everything else in the room . . . I'm going to count to 10, and as I do, let your eyes feel very heavy. Only focus on the spot and the sound of my voice. 1 . . . 2 . . . 3 . . . let your eyes feel very heavy . . . 4 . . . 5 . . . let your eyes feel heavier still . . . 6 . . . 7 . . . 8 . . . your eyes are feeling very heavy and want to close . . . 9 . . . 10 . . . let your eyes close and keep them closed.

"Very good," I said as Beth closed her eyes. "I want you to breathe very slowly, very deeply, and only pay attention to the sound of my voice. Let your whole body relax, from the top of your head all the way down to the bottoms of your feet. Let your whole body feel warm, heavy, and very relaxed. Now I want you to forget about the hospital and imagine yourself in the most beautiful park you can imagine. See the park—the grass, the hillside, a gentle brook, the beautiful trees. Hear the sounds in the park—the brook flowing, the birds singing, a light breeze rustling the leaves in the trees. Smell and taste the freshness in the air. Feel the sensations in the park—the light breeze on your skin, the warmth of the sun."

All the tension in the room evaporated.

"Now I want you to imagine a beautiful pool in the middle of the park," I continued. "It is filled with special, warm healing water. In your mind, sit on the edge of the pool and dangle your feet in it. Feel the warm water surround your feet. You are doing really great."

Beth had gone into a deep trance. I went on.

"Now I know this might sound strange, but many people can actually make their blood vessels pop up if they direct their attention to them. With your feet in the pool, allow the blood vessels in your feet to pop up so that I can put an IV in one and you can get the help you need, still allowing your mind to stay in the park and feel very relaxed."

To my great surprise, the moment I made the suggestion, a vein clearly appeared on top of Beth's swollen foot. I gently slipped the needle into the vein and attached it to the bag of IV fluid.

"Beth," I said softly, "you can stay in this deep relaxed state as long as you need. You can go back to the park anytime you want."

And with that, we wheeled a now tranquil and relaxed Beth into X-ray.

When Your Brain Works Right, You Work Right

Virtually all of us have felt anxious at some point in our lives, and that's perfectly normal. How we *respond* during these difficult times, however, can make all the difference in the world when it comes to our overall health and well-being.

Unfortunately, many people self-medicate with alcohol, drugs, overeating, or wasting time on social media. Although these things may give us temporary relief from feeling bad, they usually only prolong and often exacerbate the problems.

As a psychiatrist, a brain imaging specialist, and the founder of Amen Clinics, which has one of the highest published success rates in treating people with complex and treatment-resistant mental health issues, I can assure you that the secret to overcoming anxiety, both now and for the rest of your life, is to work on optimizing the physical functioning of your brain.

Why? Because simply put, when your brain

works right, you work right—in every area of your life. And as your brain becomes healthier, your ability to respond to everyday stressors, problems, and challenges increases exponentially, leading to fewer bouts of anxiety and better overall physical, mental, and spiritual health.

Later, I'll give you some strategies that will help you better care for your brain over the long haul (chapter 4), but first I want to walk you through some techniques (like the ones I used with Beth) to help you calm yourself down when you are in the midst of an anxiety attack or other emotional or physical crisis.

> *The secret to overcoming anxiety, both now and for the rest of your life, is to work on optimizing the physical functioning of your brain.*

Let's start by taking a closer look at how your brain and body function in a crisis. In the psychiatric profession, we call this the fight-or-flight response.

The Fight-or-Flight Stress Response

The fight-or-flight response is hardwired into our bodies to help us survive. It is mobilized into action whenever a stressor appears, such as what happened to Beth in the emergency room. Harvard physiology professor Walter Cannon first described the fight-or-flight response in 1915. He said it was the body's reaction to an acute stress, harmful event, or threat to survival, such as experiencing an earthquake or being robbed at gunpoint.

Acute stress activates the sympathetic nervous system, which prepares you to either put up a fight or flee a dangerous situation. The fight-or-flight response is triggered by the amygdala, an almond-shaped structure in the temporal lobes that is part of the limbic or emotional brain. When you become stressed, the amygdala sends a signal to the hypothalamus and pituitary gland to secrete adrenocorticotropic hormone (ACTH). This, in turn, signals the adrenal glands, on the top of the kidneys, to flood the body with cortisol, adrenaline, and other chemicals to rocket you into action.

The graphic on pages 12 and 13 illustrates what happens in our bodies when this response is set off.

The fight-or-flight response is part of a larger system in the body called the autonomic nervous system (ANS). It is called "autonomic" because its processes are largely automatic, unconscious, and out of our control, unless we train it otherwise (more on that coming up). It contains two branches that counterbalance each other: the sympathetic and parasympathetic nervous systems. Both regulate heart rate, digestion, breathing rate, pupil response, muscle tension, urination, and sexual arousal. The sympathetic nervous system (SNS) is involved in activating the fight-or-flight response, while the parasympathetic nervous system (PNS) helps to reset and calm our bodies.

Our very survival depends upon the fight-or-flight response, as it helps move us to action when there is a threat. But when stress becomes chronic, such as if you live in a war zone, grow up in an unpredictable alcoholic home, are sexually molested over time, or wake up every morning in a panic, your sympathetic nervous system becomes overactive. When that happens, you are more likely to suffer from anxiety, depression, panic attacks, headaches, cold hands and feet, breathing difficulties, high blood sugar, high blood pressure, digestive problems, immune system issues, and problems with attention and focus.

In his groundbreaking book *Why Zebras Don't Get Ulcers*, Stanford University biologist Robert Sapolsky pointed out that for animals such as zebras, stress is generally episodic (e.g., running away from a lion) and their nervous systems evolved to rapidly reset. By contrast, for humans, stress is often chronic (e.g., daily traffic, a difficult marriage, job or money worries). Sapolsky argued that many wild animals are less susceptible than humans to chronic stress-related illnesses, such as ulcers, hypertension, depression, and memory problems.[1] He did write, however, that chronic stress occurs in some primates (Dr. Sapolsky studies baboons), specifically individuals on the lower end of the social dominance hierarchy.

In humans, one big stress (such as being robbed, physically attacked, or trapped in a fire) or multiple smaller stressors (such as fighting with your spouse

THE FIGHT-OR-FLIGHT RESPONSE

Threat: an attack, harmful event, or threat to survival

Brain: processes the signals, beginning first in the amygdala and then in the hypothalamus

ACTH: pituitary gland secretes adrenocorticotropic hormone

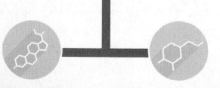

Cortisol released   Adrenaline released

PHYSICAL EFFECTS

Heart beats faster
and harder

Bladder relaxes

Pupils dilate for better
tunnel vision, but there is a
loss of peripheral vision

Erections are inhibited
(other things to
think about)

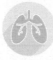

Air passages open and rapid
shallow breathing increases

Blood pressure increases

Production of tears
and saliva decreases

Digestion slows

Hearing diminishes

Muscles become tense;
trembling may occur.
Muscles around hair
follicles constrict, causing
goose bumps

Blood vessels shunt blood
to upper arms and upper
legs (fight or flee) and
away from hands and feet,
which get colder

Veins in skin constrict
(colder hands and feet) to
send more blood to major
muscle groups (to fight or
flee), causing the "chill"
sometimes associated
with fear

Blood sugar level
increases for energy

Brain has trouble focusing on
small tasks; it's thinking only
of dealing with the threat

Immune system
shuts down

or children on a regular basis) can turn on a chronic fight-or-flight state in the body, leading to mental stress and physical illness.

But by using the following techniques, you can learn to quiet your SNS and activate the PNS, which will lead you to feel calmer, happier, and less stressed.

Technique #1: Use hypnosis, guided imagery, and progressive muscle relaxation to enter a deep relaxed state.

Many people associate hypnosis with loss of control or stage tricks. But doctors know it to be a serious science, revealing the brain's ability to heal medical and psychiatric conditions.

"Hypnosis is the oldest Western form of psychotherapy, but it's been tarred with the brush of dangling watches and purple capes," said psychiatrist David Spiegel, MD, the son of a famous hypnotist and associate chair of psychiatry and behavioral sciences at Stanford University School of Medicine. "In fact, it's a very powerful means of changing the way we use our minds to control perception and our bodies. . . . The power of hypnosis to immediately change your brain is real."[2]

Using hypnosis, guided imagery, or progressive muscle relaxation (PMR) increases parasympathetic tone and can quickly decrease the fight-or-flight response in a wide variety of conditions, as it did for Beth. These techniques have been found to have many benefits, including lowering anxiety, sadness, and tension in parents of children with cancer;[3] pain and fatigue in those receiving chemotherapy;[4] stress in those with multiple sclerosis;[5] anxiety and depression;[6] migraine frequency;[7] tension headaches;[8] craving and withdrawal symptoms in people quitting smoking;[9] post-stroke anxiety (a result of listening to a PMR CD five times a week);[10] and phantom limb pain.[11] They can also improve quality of life in the elderly[12] and dialysis patients,[13] fatigue in the elderly, and sexual function in postmenopausal women.[14]

Learning hypnosis, guided imagery, and progressive muscle relaxation is simple; there are many online audios that can guide you. We have several on our Brain Fit Life site (www.mybrainfitlife.com). You can certainly do it yourself. Below are the instructions I give my patients to help them go into a deep relaxed state. The skill builds over time, so it is important to practice this exercise to gain mastery. Set aside two 15-minute periods a day and go through the following five steps:

1. Sit in a comfortable chair with your feet on the floor and your hands in your lap. Pick a spot on the opposite wall that is a little bit above your eye level. Stare at the spot. As you do, slowly count

to 20. Notice that your eyelids soon begin to feel heavy, as if they want to close. Let them. In fact, even if they don't feel as if they want to close, slowly lower them as you get to 20.

2. Take a deep breath, as deep as you can, and very slowly exhale. Repeat the deep breath and slow exhale three times. With each in-breath, imagine taking in peace and calmness, and with each out-breath, blow out all the tension—all the things getting in the way of your relaxing. By this time, you'll notice a calm come over you.

3. Squeeze the muscles in your eyelids, closing your eyes as tightly as you can. Then slowly let the muscles in your eyelids relax. Imagine that relaxation slowly spreading, like a warm, penetrating oil, from the muscles in your eyelids to the muscles in your face—down your neck, into your shoulders and arms, into your chest, and throughout the rest of your body. The muscles will take the cue from your eyelids and relax progressively all the way down to the bottoms of your feet.

4. When all the tension has left your body, imagine yourself at the top of an escalator. Step on the escalator and ride down, counting backward from 10. By the time you reach the bottom, you'll be very relaxed.

5. Enjoy the tranquility for several moments. Then get back on the escalator riding up, counting to 10 as you go. When you get to 10, open your eyes, feeling relaxed, refreshed, and wide-awake.

   To make these steps easy to remember, think of the following words:

   - **Focus** (focus on the spot)
   - **Breathe** (slow, deep breaths)
   - **Relax** (progressive muscle relaxation)
   - **Down** (ride down the escalator)
   - **Up** (ride up the escalator and open your eyes)

If you have trouble remembering these steps, you may want to record them as you read them aloud and then do the exercise as you listen to the audio.

Allow yourself plenty of time to do this. Some people become so relaxed that they fall asleep for several minutes. If that happens, don't worry. It's a good sign—you're really relaxed!

Once you've practiced this technique a few times, add the following steps:

1. Choose a haven—a place where you feel comfortable and that you can imagine with all your senses. I usually "go" to the beach. I can see the ocean, feel the sand between my toes and the warm sun

and breeze on my skin, smell the salt air and taste it faintly on my tongue, and hear the seagulls, the waves, and children playing. Your haven can be any real or imaginary place where you'd like to spend time.

2. After you reach the bottom of the escalator, use all your senses to imagine yourself in your special haven. Stay for several minutes. This is where the fun starts and where your mind becomes ripe for change.

3. Begin to experience yourself—not as you currently are, but as you *want* to be. Plan on spending at least 20 minutes a day on this refueling, life-changing exercise. You'll be amazed at the results.

Technique #2: Master diaphragmatic breathing.

In the chapter's opening story, the first thing I did with Beth was help her to slow her breathing so she could get more oxygen to her brain. Diaphragmatic breathing is a core biofeedback technique to help you feel better fast. It is simple to teach and, once practiced, simple to implement and maintain.

Like brain activity, breathing is essential to life and involved in everything you do. Breathing delivers oxygen from the atmosphere into your lungs, where your bloodstream picks it up and takes it to all of the cells in your body so that they can function properly. Breathing also allows you to eliminate waste products, such as carbon dioxide, which can cause feelings of disorientation and panic. Brain cells are particularly sensitive to oxygen; within four minutes of being deprived of it, they start to die. Slight changes in oxygen content in the brain can alter the way you feel and behave.

BREATHING ANATOMY

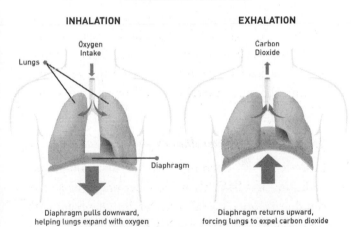

INHALATION

Oxygen Intake

Lungs

Diaphragm

Diaphragm pulls downward, helping lungs expand with oxygen

EXHALATION

Carbon Dioxide

Diaphragm returns upward, forcing lungs to expel carbon dioxide

The diaphragm, a bell-shaped muscle, separates the chest cavity from the abdomen. Many people never flatten the diaphragm when they inhale, and thus with each breath they have less access to their own lung capacity and have to work harder. By moving your belly out when you inhale, you flatten the diaphragm, significantly increase lung capacity, and calm all body systems.

When someone gets angry or anxious, their breathing becomes shallow and fast (see the "Breathing Anatomy" diagram on page 19). This causes the oxygen in an angry person's blood to decrease, while toxic carbon dioxide increases. Subsequently, the oxygen/carbon dioxide balance is upset, causing irritability, impulsiveness, confusion, and bad decision-making.

Learning how to direct and control your breathing has several immediate benefits. It calms the amygdala (part of the emotional brain), counteracts the fight-or-flight response, relaxes muscles, warms hands, and regulates the heart's rhythms. I often teach patients to become experts at breathing slowly, deeply, and from their bellies. If you watch babies or puppies, you will notice that they breathe almost solely with their bellies—the most efficient way to breathe.

Expanding your belly when you inhale flattens the diaphragm, pulling the lungs downward and increasing the amount of air available to your lungs and body. Pulling your belly in when you exhale causes the diaphragm to push the air out of your lungs, allowing for a more fully exhaled breath, which once again encourages deep breathing. In biofeedback, patients are taught to breathe with their bellies by watching their breathing pattern on the computer screen. In 20 to 30 minutes, most people can learn how to change their breathing patterns, which relaxes them and gives them better control over how they feel and behave.

BREATHING DURING ANGER

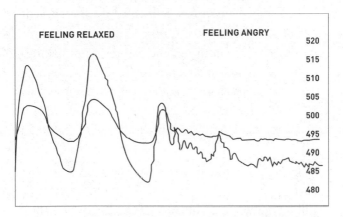

The large waveform is a measurement of abdominal or belly breathing, by a strain gauge attached around the belly; the smaller waveform is a measurement of chest breathing, by a strain gauge attached around the upper chest. At rest, this person breathes mostly with his belly (a good pattern), but when he thinks about an angry situation his breathing pattern deteriorates, markedly decreasing the oxygen to his brain (common to anger outbursts). No wonder people who have anger outbursts often seem irrational!

Controlled diaphragmatic breathing has been shown to improve focus and lower anxiety, stress, negative feelings, and cortisol;[15] decrease depression[16] and asthma;[17] reduce obesity in children,[18] pain,[19] blood pressure,[20] motion sickness,[21] and seizure frequency;[22] and boost the quality of life in heart failure patients.[23]

Breathing Techniques to Help You Calm Down Fast

Breathing Technique #1: While few people have access to sophisticated biofeedback equipment, these simple techniques can be effective for everyone. Try the following exercise right now: Lie on your back and place a small book on your belly. When you inhale, make the book rise by expanding your belly; when you exhale, pull your belly in, which will lower the book. Shifting the energy of breathing lower in your body—from your upper chest into your abdomen—will help you feel more relaxed and in better control of yourself almost instantaneously. Practice this for five minutes every day until it feels natural. You can use this breathing technique to gain greater focus and control over your temper. It is easy to learn, and it can also help with sleep and anxiety issues.

Breathing Technique #2: Whenever you feel anxious, mad, or tense, take a deep breath, hold it for one or two seconds, and then slowly exhale for about five seconds. Then take another deep breath, as deep as you can, hold it for one to two seconds, and again slowly exhale. Do this about 10 times, and odds are that you will start to feel very relaxed, if not a little sleepy. I have used this technique myself for 30 years whenever I feel anxious, angry, or stressed, or when I have trouble falling asleep. It sounds so simple, but breathing is essential to life. When we slow down and become more efficient with our breathing, most things seem better.

Technique #3: Become expert at warming your hands with your mind.

Visualizing warmth, especially in your hands, is another tool to help you counteract the fight-or-flight response. I've found that teaching patients to warm their hands calms down their bodies and minds just as effectively as prescription drugs. Hand warming elicits an immediate relaxation response. We know this because biofeedback instruments allow us to measure hand temperature and then teach people how to warm their hands. Interestingly, children are better at this than adults because kids readily believe they have power over their bodies, whereas adults do not.

When my daughter Breanne was eight years old, she could increase her hand temperature by up to 20 degrees. She was so good at it, I brought her along with me when I did a biofeedback lecture to physicians at a Northern California hospital. In front of 30 physicians, I had her demonstrate her amazing skill. However, for the first three minutes her hands did nothing but get ice-cold because she felt such performance anxiety. In those few minutes I was horrified, feeling like a terrible father who was exploiting his daughter to be important in front of his colleagues. Then I whispered in her ear that she should close her eyes, take a deep breath, and imagine her hands in the warm sand at the beach (the image that worked best for her). Over the next seven minutes, her hands warmed 18 degrees. The doctors were amazed, she was so happy with herself, and I was relieved that I had not scarred her for life.

How can you warm your hands with your mind? You do it with diaphragmatic breathing and the visualization that works for you. For some, like Breanne, it's imagining putting your hands in warm sand at the beach. For others, it's thinking about holding a loved one's hand or touching their warm skin. For still others, it's visualizing holding a warm, furry kitten or puppy.

Let's try it. Take a moment to focus on your hands, feeling their energy and temperature. Now close your eyes and hold out your hands, palms down, and visualize a campfire in front of you. Focus. Think heat. You can hear the fire crackle, smell the aroma of fresh-cut wood burning, see the sparks float up into the sky. Now feel the soothing heat as it penetrates the surface of your skin and goes deep to warm your hands. Picture this as you breathe deeply and count slowly to 20.

Did you feel an increase in warmth? Relaxation?

Did you find you started to hold your hands closer as if there were actually a fire in front of you?

Practice this technique for a few minutes every day, and you'll find you get to the relaxation response more easily and faster over time. Find the hand-warming images that work for you, and you will reset your nervous system to be more relaxed and counteract your stress response. You can buy temperature sensors online (under brand names Biodots, Stress Cards, and Stress Sheets) to get feedback on your progress.

---

13 Hand-Warming Images

1. Holding someone's warm hand or touching their warm skin

2. Visualizing (in great detail) someone you appreciate

3. Putting your hands in warm sand at the beach

4. Taking a hot bath or shower

5. Sitting in a sauna

6. Cuddling a baby

7. Cuddling a warm, furry puppy or kitten

8. Holding a warm cup of tea or sugar-free cocoa

9. Holding your hands in front of a fire

10. Wearing warm gloves

11. Being wrapped in a warm towel

12. Getting a massage with warm oil

13. Holding a hot potato while wearing warm gloves

Technique #4: Pray and/or practice meditation (especially Loving-Kindness Meditation).

Focusing on your breathing, a beautiful outdoor scene, or Scripture for just five to ten minutes a day is a simple yet powerful way not only to help quell anxious thoughts but also to improve your life overall. Prayer and meditation have been found to calm stress; improve focus, mood, and memory; and enhance prefrontal cortex function to help you make better decisions. What's more, meditation benefits your heart and blood pressure, digestion, and immune system, as well as improves executive function and emotional control and reduces feelings of anxiety, depression, and irritability.[24]

Prayer and meditation have been found to calm stress; improve focus, mood, and memory; and enhance prefrontal cortex function to help you make better decisions.

There are many effective techniques, including reading, memorizing, or meditating on Scripture; writing out a personal prayer; reading classic spiritual writings; or focusing on gratitude. One of my personal favorite forms of meditation is called Loving-Kindness Meditation (LKM), which is intended to develop feelings of goodwill and warmth toward others. It has been found to quickly increase positive emotions and decrease negative ones,[25] decrease pain[26] and migraine headaches,[27] reduce symptoms of post-traumatic stress disorder[28] and social prejudice,[29] increase gray matter in the emotional processing areas of the brain,[30] and boost social connectedness.[31] Here's how it works.

Sit in a comfortable and relaxed position and close your eyes. Take two or three deep breaths, taking twice as long to exhale as inhale. Let any worries or concerns drift away, and feel your breath moving through the area around your heart. As you sit, quietly or silently repeat the following or similar phrases:

> May I be safe and secure.
> May I be healthy and strong.
> May I be happy and purposeful.
> May I be at peace.

Let the intentions expressed in these phrases sink in as you repeat them. Allow the feelings to grow deeper.

After a few repetitions, direct the phrases to someone you feel grateful for or someone who has helped you:

May you be safe and secure.
May you be healthy and strong.
May you be happy and purposeful.
May you be at peace.

Next visualize someone you feel neutral about. Choose among people you neither like nor dislike and repeat the phrases.

Now visualize someone you don't like or with whom you are having a hard time and repeat the phrases with that person in mind. Kids who are being teased or bullied at school often feel quite empowered when they send love to the people who are making them miserable.

Finally, direct the phrases more broadly: *May everyone be safe and secure.*

You can do this for up to 30 minutes; it is up to you.

Technique #5: Create your emotional rescue playlist.

Music can soothe, inspire, improve your mood, and help you focus. It is important in every known culture on earth, with ancient roots extending back thousands of years.[32] After evaluating more than 800 people, researchers have found that people listen to music to regulate their energy and mood, to achieve self-awareness, and to improve social bonds. Music provides social cement—think of work and war songs, lullabies, and national anthems.[33] In his powerful book *The Secret Language of the Heart*, Barry Goldstein reviewed the neuroscientific properties of music. He suggested that music stimulates emotional circuits in the brain[34] and releases oxytocin, the "cuddle hormone," which can enhance bonding, trust, and relationships.[35] He wrote, "Listening to music can create peak emotions, which increase the amount of dopamine, a specific neurotransmitter that is produced in the brain and helps control the brain's reward and pleasure centers. . . . Music was used to assist patients with severe brain injuries in recalling personal memories. The music helped the patients to reconnect to memories they previously could not access."[36] Be aware, however, that music you strongly like or dislike may impair your focus.[37]

Based on the concept of entrainment, which means your brain picks up the rhythm of your environment, you can manipulate your mind with the music you choose. In a fascinating study, research subjects rated Mozart's Sonata for Two Pianos (K. 448) and Beethoven's Moonlight Sonata as happy and sad, respectively.[38] Listening to happy music (Mozart's piece) increased activity in the brain's left hemisphere, associated with happiness and motivation, and decreased activity in the right hemisphere, often associated with anxiety and negativity. Beethoven's piece did the opposite.

According to research published in the *Journal of Positive Psychology*, you can improve your mood and boost your overall happiness in just two weeks, simply by having the intention of being happier and by listening to specific mood-boosting music, such as Aaron Copland's *Rodeo*, for 12 minutes a day.[39] Having only the intention to be happier was not as effective. Listening to happy instrumental music (versus music with lyrics) was more powerful in activating the limbic or emotional circuits of the brain.[40]

Create your own emotional rescue playlist to boost your mood quickly. Research shows it can be effective to start with musical pieces you love. If you're not sure where to start, try some of these pieces, which have been shown through research to boost mood:

Without lyrics (words can be distracting[41]):
- Sonata for Two Pianos in D Major, third movement (K. 448) – Mozart (~ 6 min.)
- "Clair de Lune" – Debussy (~ 5 min.)
- "Adagio for Strings" – Samuel Barber (~ 8 min.)
- Piano Sonata no. 17 in D Minor ("The Tempest") – Beethoven (~ 25 min.)
- "First Breath after Coma" – Explosions in the Sky (9:33 min.)
- "Adagio for Strings" – Tiësto (9:34 original; 7:23 album version)
- "Fanfare for the Common Man" – Aaron Copland (~ 4 min.)

- "Weightless" – Marconi Union (8:09 min.)
- "Flotus" – Flying Lotus (3:27 min.)
- "Lost in Thought" – Jon Hopkins (6:16 min.)
- "The Soundmaker" – Rodrigo y Gabriela (4:54 min.)
- "See" – Tycho (5:18 min.)
- "Spectre" – Tycho (3:47 min.)

Add nature sounds (your own recordings or downloads of favorites) to boost mood and focus.[42]

With lyrics:[43]

- "Good Vibrations" – The Beach Boys (3:16 min.)
- "Don't Stop Me Now" – Queen (3:36 min.)
- "Uptown Girl" – Billy Joel (3:23 min.)
- "Dancing Queen" – ABBA (3:45 min.)
- "Eye of the Tiger" – Survivor (4:11 min.)
- "I'm a Believer" – The Monkees (2:46 min.)
- "Girls Just Want to Have Fun" – Cyndi Lauper (4:25 min.)
- "Livin' on a Prayer" – Bon Jovi (4:09 min.)
- "I Will Survive" – Gloria Gaynor (3:11 min.)
- "Walking on Sunshine" – Katrina and the Waves (3:48 min.)

Brain-enhancing music specifically composed by Barry Goldstein to enhance creativity, mood, memory, gratitude, energy, focus, motivation, and inspiration can be found at www.mybrainfitlife.com. Treat your brain and listen often.

Technique #6: Flood your five senses with positivity.

The brain senses the world. If you can change the inputs, you can often quickly change how you feel.

Hearing: As we have just seen, music can help to optimize your state of being.

Touch: Positive touch is powerful. Getting a hug, a massage, acupuncture, or acupressure or spending time in a sauna can improve mood. Massage has been shown to improve pain, mood, and anxiety in fibromyalgia patients;[44] mood and pain in cancer patients;[45] and mood after open-heart surgery.[46] It has also been shown to improve mood and behavior in students with ADHD.[47] Likewise, acupuncture and acupressure can help with premenstrual syndrome (PMS),[48] depression,[49] anxiety and anger,[50] and pain.[51] Saunas have been shown to enhance mood after just one session,[52] increase

> *The brain senses the world. If you can change the inputs, you can often quickly change how you feel.*

endorphins (feel-good chemicals),[53] and decrease the risk of Alzheimer's disease.[54]

Smell: Certain scents are known to have positive effects on how we feel, especially lavender oil (for anxiety,[55] mood,[56] sleep,[57] and migraine headaches[58]), rose oil,[59] and chamomile.[60]

Sight: Soothing images can impact your mood. Images of nature[61] and fractals (never-ending patterns)[62] can soothe stress. In one study, people who looked at real plants or posters of plants experienced less stress while waiting for medical procedures.[63]

Taste: Flavoring food with cinnamon, saffron, mint, sage, or nutmeg has been shown to enhance mood.[64]

A fun way to put this all together to change your state of mind might be to take a sauna while listening to "Good Vibrations" and watching scenes of the ocean, all with the scent of lavender or rose oil in the air and while sipping on a cinnamon almond-milk cappuccino!

These six techniques are effective ways to help you feel better fast when you're anxious or upset. Come back to them anytime you need to regain control over your mind and body.

CHAPTER 2

HOW TO FEEL HAPPY AND PRESENT

Conquering Worry and Negativity

A thought is harmless unless we believe it. It's not our thoughts, but the attachment *to our thoughts, that causes suffering. Attaching to a thought means believing that it's true, without inquiring. A belief is a thought that we've been attaching to, often for years.*

BYRON KATIE, *LOVING WHAT IS:*
FOUR QUESTIONS THAT CAN CHANGE YOUR LIFE

Dark thoughts in the mind are not "you," but are false messages from the brain. And because you are not your brain, you don't have to listen to them.

JEFFREY M. SCHWARTZ, MD,
AUTHOR OF *YOU ARE NOT YOUR BRAIN*

Now that we've talked about a few ways to help you calm down during a crisis, let's turn our attention to maintaining your emotional center from day to day. Like anything else—losing weight, mastering a sport, or learning to play a musical instrument—it all comes down to discipline.

Developing the habit of accurate, honest, and disciplined thinking is essential to overcoming worry and anxiety.

Now, this is *not* positive thinking, which can actually inhibit feeling better over the long run. People who live by the philosophy "Don't worry; be happy" tend to die the earliest from accidents and preventable illnesses. Why? Because believing the future will be favorable without following a plan and putting in consistent effort can prevent people from taking the actions that will likely make that belief a reality.[1]

This chapter will help you develop the mental discipline necessary for success, including eliminating the ANTs (automatic negative thoughts), quieting your mind, having an appropriate level of anxiety, and focusing on gratitude.

You Are What You Think

According to a 2015 study from Microsoft, the human attention span is eight seconds.[2] To give you a little perspective, a goldfish's attention span has been estimated at nine seconds. Simply put, human development seems to be going the wrong way, and the technology we were led to believe is helping us is actually making it worse![3] Studies show that people who have the most screen time (TV, texting, video games) have a higher incidence of feeling unhappy.

With modern technology stealing our attention span and directing our minds to the will of corporate

America, disciplining the habits of our moment-by-moment thoughts is an essential skill for achieving and maintaining happiness and purpose.

Every time you have a thought, your brain releases chemicals. That's how your brain works. You have a thought, your brain releases chemicals, electrical transmissions travel throughout your brain, and you become aware of what you're thinking. Thoughts are real, and they have a powerful impact on how you feel and behave. Just as a muscle that's exercised becomes stronger, repeatedly thinking the same thoughts makes them stronger too.

Every time you have an angry, unkind, hopeless, helpless, worthless, sad, or irritating thought, such as *I'm stupid*, your brain releases chemicals that make you feel bad. In this way, your body reacts to every negative thought you have. When most people are angry, their muscles become tense, their hearts beat faster, their hands start to sweat, and they may even begin to feel a little dizzy.

Similarly, every time you have a happy, hopeful, kind, optimistic, positive thought, your brain releases chemicals that make you feel good. When most people are happy, their muscles relax, their hearts beat more slowly, their hands become dry, and they breathe more evenly.

Your body reacts to every thought you have, whether it is about work, friends, family, or anything else. This is why when people become upset, they often develop physical symptoms, such as headaches, stomachaches, or diarrhea, or they become more susceptible to illness. Just as pollution in Los Angeles or Beijing affects everyone who goes outdoors, so, too, do negative thoughts pollute your mind and your body.

In generations past, negative thoughts protected us from early death or becoming supper for powerful animals, so in essence, being aware of and avoiding danger was crucial to survival. Unfortunately, even when the world became safer, negativity bias remained in our brains.

Researchers have demonstrated that negative experiences have a greater impact on the brain than positive ones.[4] People pay more attention to negative than to positive news, which is why news outlets typically lead broadcasts with floods, murders, political disasters, and all forms of mayhem. According to research from the content marketing website Outbrain.com, in two periods of 2012 the average click-through rate on headlines with negative adjectives was an astounding 63 percent higher than for headlines with positive ones.[5] Unfortunately, a negative perspective is more contagious than a positive one, which may be why political campaigns typically go negative at the end.

Even our language is not exempt: 62 percent of the words in the English dictionary connote negative emotions, while only 32 percent express positive ones.[6]

Psychologist and author Rick Hanson has written that the brain is wired for negativity bias. Bad news is quickly stored in the brain to keep us safe, but positive experiences have to be held in consciousness for more than 12 seconds before they stay with us. "The brain is like Velcro for negative experiences but Teflon for positive ones," Hanson wrote.[7]

Further, psychologist Mihaly Csikszentmihalyi, author of *Flow: The Psychology of Optimal Experience*, suggested that without other thoughts to occupy us, our brains will always return to worry. The only way to escape this is to focus on what will bring "flow"— activities that increase our sense of purpose and achievement.

In short, negative emotions "trump" positive emotions, which is why it is critical to discipline your natural tendency toward the negative and amplify more helpful thoughts and emotions. Unless disciplined and bridled, negative thoughts (*I am worthless; I am stupid; I have no control over anything in my life*) will lie to you and wreak havoc in your life. If you never challenge your thoughts, you will simply believe them and then act out of that erroneous belief.

If, for example, I thought, *My wife never listens to me*, I'd feel lonely, mad, and sad. I would give myself permission to be rude to her or ignore her. My reaction to the lie I was telling myself could cause a negative spiral in my marriage, which could then literally ruin the rest of my life.

By repeatedly allowing undisciplined thoughts to invade your mind, you are more likely to behave in ways that make terrible things happen, which is why it is critical to get control over your thoughts.

Conquering the Negative Thoughts That Steal Your Happiness

I coined the term *ANTs* in the early 1990s after a hard day at the office. I had seen four suicidal patients, two teens who had run away from home, and two couples who hated each other, and then that evening, when I arrived home and walked into the kitchen, I was greeted by an ant infestation. There were thousands of the pesky invaders marching in lines on the floor and crawling in the sink, on the countertops, and in the cabinets. Construction in our neighborhood had disturbed the earth, and the ants were looking for a new residence. As I wetted paper towels and began wiping up the horde of ants, the acronym ANT— automatic negative thought—just came to me.

As I thought about my patients that day, I realized that, just like my kitchen, they were also infested with ANTs that were robbing them of their joy and stealing their happiness, and a bizarre image came to me of ANTs crawling on top of their heads and out of their eyes, noses, and ears. The ANTs were literally setting up residence inside my patients' minds. The next day, I brought a can of ant spray to work and placed it on my coffee table. As I started to talk about the concept with my patients, they understood it right away.

Think of automatic negative thoughts as you would the ants that might bother a couple at a romantic picnic. One negative thought, like one ant at a picnic, is not a big problem. Two or three automatic negative thoughts, like two or three ants at a picnic, become a bit more irritating. Twenty or thirty automatic negative thoughts, like twenty or thirty ants at a picnic, may cause the couple to pick up and leave. The more you allow the ANTs to stick around in your head, the more they will "mate" with other ANTs and produce offspring that drive anxiety, depression, anger, and relationship turmoil.

ANTs are thoughts that pop into your mind uninvited. They make you feel mad, sad, worried, or upset. And most of the time they're not even true!

As the discussions about ANTs continued in my office, I eventually replaced the can of ant spray with a black ant puppet and an adorable, furry anteater puppet. I then developed a simple exercise to help my patients eliminate the ANTs: *Whenever you feel sad, mad, nervous, or out of control, write down your automatic negative thoughts and talk back to them.* When you have a negative thought without challenging it (*I'm worthless*), your mind believes it and your body reacts to it. But, if you can correct negative thoughts (*I was made in the image of God. I bring value and joy to my spouse's life, my children's lives, and my friends' lives*), you take away their power.

Learning how to direct, question, and correct your automatic negative thoughts is not a new concept. Two of my favorite New Testament verses are from the apostle Paul:

> Whatever is true, whatever is noble,
> whatever is right, whatever is pure, whatever
> is lovely, whatever is admirable—if anything
> is excellent or praiseworthy—think about
> such things.
> PHILIPPIANS 4:8, NIV

> Be transformed by the renewing of your
> mind.
> ROMANS 12:2, NIV

Even 2,000 years ago, Paul taught about the benefits of filling our minds with what is good and positive! And more recently, in the 1960s, psychiatrist Aaron Beck formalized a school of psychotherapy called cognitive behavioral therapy (CBT), which is a structured way to teach patients to challenge and eliminate negative thoughts.

The good news is, you *can* learn how to eliminate

the automatic negative thoughts and replace them with more helpful thoughts that give you a more accurate, fair assessment of any situation. And it's not just "positive thinking" that ignores reality; it is accurate, honest thinking, and once you learn how to do it, it can completely change your life.

Over the years, therapists have identified seven different types of negative thought patterns that keep your mind off-balance. I like to think of these as "species" of ANTs. They go by various names, but the ones I like to use are:

1. **All-or-Nothing ANTs:** Thinking that things are either all good or all bad
2. **Just the Bad ANTs:** Seeing only the bad in a situation
3. **Guilt-Beating ANTs:** Thinking in words like *should, must, ought,* or *have to*
4. **Labeling ANTs:** Attaching a negative label to yourself or someone else
5. **Fortune-Teller ANTs:** Predicting the worst possible outcome for a situation with little or no evidence for it
6. **Mind Reader ANTs:** Believing you know what other people are thinking even though they haven't told you
7. **Blaming ANTs:** Blaming someone else for your problems

Let's take a closer look at each and talk about ways you can stomp them out once and for all.

1. **All-or-Nothing ANTs.** These sneaky ANTs make you feel sorry for yourself. They don't use words like *sometimes* or *maybe*. All-or-Nothing ANTs think in absolutes—words like *all, always, never, none, nothing, no one, everyone,* and *every time*.

   I once met a woman who told me she hated the gym so much that she would never exercise. This is an example of all-or-nothing thinking, believing that everything is either *all* good or *all* bad. The key to overcoming All-or-Nothing ANTs is to stop thinking in absolute terms.

   "Do you like to dance?" I asked her.

   "Oh, I love to dance," she replied.

   "How about taking a walk on the beach?" I asked.

   "I like that too," she said.

   When I told her that dancing and walking on the beach are forms of exercise, she gave me a puzzled look. She had always equated "exercise" with the gym. When she realized that *any* type of physical activity qualified as exercise, she said, "Maybe I don't hate to exercise; maybe I just hate the gym."

   Questioning the ANTs helps to send them packing.

2. **Just the Bad ANTs.** This ANT can't see anything good! Its beady eyes zoom in on mistakes and problems, and it fills your head with failure, frustration, sadness, and fear. As we discussed earlier, the brain is wired for negativity, and this ANT can take virtually *any* positive experience and taint it with negativity. It is the judge, jury, and executioner of new experiences, new relationships, and new habits.

   Some examples of Just the Bad ANTs include thoughts like these:

   I wanted to lose 30 pounds in 10 weeks, but I've only lost 8 pounds. I'm a complete failure.

   I went to the gym and did a hard workout, but the guy on the bike next to me was talking the whole time, so I'm never going back there.

   I gave a presentation at work to 30 people. Even though people told me they liked it, one person fell asleep during my talk, so it must have really been terrible.

   As we've seen, focusing on the negative releases brain chemicals that make you feel bad, and that reduces brain activity in the area involved with self-control, judgment, and planning. This, in turn, increases the odds of your making bad choices, such as ordering a third drink, eating a bowlful of chips, or staying up so late updating your social networking site that you wake up exhausted and need to guzzle caffeine to get going.

> *Putting a positive spin on your thoughts leads to positive changes in your brain that make you happier and smarter.*

But just as focusing on Just the Bad ANTs sets you up for failure, focusing on the *positive* will improve your mood and help you feel better about yourself. Putting a positive spin on your thoughts leads to positive changes in your brain that make you happier and smarter. Here's how one could think differently about those situations listed above:

> *I have already lost 8 pounds and have changed my lifestyle, so I will continue to lose weight until I reach my goal of losing 30 pounds.*

> *After working out, I had a lot more energy for the rest of the day.*

> *Most people told me they liked my presentation. I wonder if the person who fell asleep during it stayed up too late last night.*

3. **Guilt-Beating ANTs.** Growing up Roman Catholic and going to parochial schools through ninth grade, I had to pass both Guilt 101 and Advanced Guilt. Just kidding—but *should* and *shouldn't* were both common words when I was growing up. Of course, there are many important *should* and *shouldn't* thoughts (*you shouldn't overeat*; *you shouldn't drink to excess*), but in my more than 35 years as a psychiatrist, I've found that guilt is generally *not* a helpful motivator of behavior, as it often backfires and can be counterproductive to your goals.

   Here are some examples of Guilt-Beating ANTs:

   I should visit my parents.

   I have to give up sugar.

   I must start counting my calories.

   I ought to go to the gym more.

   I should be more giving.

   What happens when you allow these ANTs to circle in your mind? Do they make you more inclined to visit your parents, cut the sugar, count calories, hit the gym, or be more giving? I doubt it. It is human nature to push back when we feel as if we "must" do something, even if it is to our benefit.

The key to overcoming Guilt-Beating ANTs is to replace them with phrases like *I want to do this, It fits with my goals to do that*, or *It would be helpful to do this*. Following this line of thinking, it would be beneficial to change the phrases in the examples above:

> *I want to visit my parents because they are special to me.*

> *My goal is to stop eating sugar because it will reduce my cravings; prevent energy crashes, diabetes, and inflammation in my body; and get me off this emotional roller coaster.*

> *I want to count my calories because it will help me learn to take control of my eating.*

> *It is in my best interest to go to the gym because it will help me feel more energized.*

> *I am a giving person, and it is my goal to give more to causes I believe are worthwhile.*

4. **Labeling ANTs.** Whenever you label yourself or someone else with a negative term, you inhibit your ability to take an honest look at the situation. Labeling ANTs strengthen negative

pathways in the brain, making the ruts deeper and their walls thicker. These habitual ruts lead to troubled behaviors. If, for example, you label yourself as "lazy," then why bother trying to do better in school or at work? Labeling ANTs will cause you to give up before you try, and they will keep you stuck in your old ways. Examples of Labeling ANTs include:

I'm lazy.

I'm a loser.

I'm a lousy businessperson.

The problem with Labeling ANTs is that they trick you into thinking that it is impossible to change. You are what you are. But that's not true! Remember, Paul tells us that we can be transformed by the renewing of our minds. So change your thinking to focus on what's possible:

I know I can do better in school if I just apply myself more. I'm going to ask my teacher to help me set up a study plan and show me some time-management skills.

I am capable of so much more than I have given myself credit for. I am going to commit to eating better, exercising more, and spending more time with family and friends.

I know I can do better at work. I'm going to make a list of my strengths and strategize ways to use them more effectively.

A word of caution: Even positive labels can be harmful. I tell parents, for example, never to praise children for being smart; praise them instead for working hard. When you tell children they are smart, they become more performance oriented and assume that intelligence cannot be improved. If they start to struggle with a new task, they may feel "not smart" and give up. But if you praise children for working hard, when they come up against a difficult task, they will persist because "they work hard."

5. **Fortune-Teller ANTs.** Don't listen to these lying ANTs! Fortune-Teller ANTs think they can see what is going to happen in the future, but all they really do is think up bad stuff that makes you upset. They creep into your mind and fill the future with fear. Of course, it is always helpful to prepare for potential problems, but if you spend all your time focused on a fearful future, you will be filled with anxiety. Examples of this deceiver include:

If I run, I'll sprain my ankle.

If I give that presentation, I will have a panic attack.

None of my investments will pay off.

If I go to bed earlier, I'm just going to lie there awake for hours.

Predicting the worst in a situation causes an immediate rise in heart and breathing rates and can make you feel anxious. It can trigger cravings for sugar or refined carbs and make you feel as if you need to eat to calm your anxiety.

What makes Fortune-Teller ANTs even worse is that your mind is so powerful, it can make what you imagine happen. When you think you will sprain your ankle, for example, that thought may deactivate the cerebellum, making you more clumsy and likely to get hurt. Similarly, if you are convinced you won't get a good night's sleep or find a new relationship, you will be less likely to engage in the behaviors that might make it so.

The key to eliminating this ANT is to talk back to it:

As long as I stretch and remain focused when I run, I will be fine.

I am going to ace that presentation.

I am going to make sound, informed financial investments. That way, even if some of them don't work out, I'll still land on my feet.

If I can't fall asleep right away, I'll just read a good book until I get tired.

6. **Mind Reader ANTs.** This ANT is convinced it can see inside someone else's mind and know how others think and feel without even being told. It leads you to tell yourself things like, *Everyone thinks I am stupid* or *They are laughing at me.* When you're sure you know what others are thinking even though they have not told you and you have not asked them, you are feeding your Mind Reader ANTs.

I have 25 years of education, and I can't tell what anyone else is thinking unless they tell me. A glance in your direction doesn't mean somebody is talking about you or mad at you. I tell people that a negative look from someone else may mean nothing more than that he or she is constipated! You just don't know. Other examples of Mind Reader ANTs include thoughts like:

My boss doesn't like me.

My martial arts teacher doesn't respect me because I'm fat.

My friends think I won't be able to keep up with them on our hike.

My father thinks I'll never amount to much.

I teach all my patients the "18-40-60 Rule," which says that when you are 18 you worry about what everyone thinks of you; when you are 40 you don't care what anyone thinks about you; and when you are 60 you realize no one has been thinking about you at all. The vast majority of people spend their days worrying and thinking about themselves, not about you, so stop trying to read their minds. Don't let this ANT erase your good feelings. When there are things you don't understand, ask for clarification. Mind Reader ANTs are infectious and cause trouble between people.

> *The vast majority of people spend their days worrying and thinking about themselves, not about you, so stop trying to read their minds.*

7. **Blaming ANTs.** When things go wrong, the Blaming ANT always sings the same old sad song: *He did it! She did it! It's not my fault! It's your fault!* This ANT doesn't want you to admit

your mistakes or to learn how to fix things and make them right; it wants you to be a victim.

Of all the ANTs, Blaming ANTs are the most toxic. I call them red ANTs, because they not only steal your happiness, they also drain you of your personal power. When you blame something or someone else for the problems in your life, you become a victim of circumstances who can't do anything to change the situation. Be honest with yourself. Ask yourself if you have a tendency to say things like:

If only you hadn't done that, I would have been successful.

It's your fault I failed because you didn't do enough to help me.

It's not my fault I eat too much; my mom taught me to clean my plate.

I'm having trouble meeting this deadline because the client keeps changing his mind. I'm miserable, and it's all his fault!

My boyfriend didn't call on time, and now it's too late to go to that movie I wanted to see. He's ruined my night!

Beginning a sentence with "It is *your* fault that I . . ." can ruin your life. In order to break free from the Blaming ANT addiction, you have to change your thinking by making it your responsibility to change. It is your life.

I love what author Vernon Howard once wrote: "Permitting your life to be taken over by another person is like letting the waiter eat your dinner."

At the same time, self-blame is equally toxic. Always strive to be a good coach to yourself, rather than someone who is toxic or abusive.

As you can see, it is possible to learn how to listen to your thoughts and redirect them so that you feel happier and more positive. Whenever you feel sad, mad, nervous, or out of control:

1. Write down your automatic negative thoughts (ANTs).
2. Identify the ANT species. (It may be more than one.)
3. Ask yourself if you are 100 percent sure the thought is true.
4. Redirect your thoughts to focus on what *is* true.

Confronting ANTs with truth is a powerful tool. Don't believe every stupid thought you have. Instead, remember the wisdom of Paul: "Whatever is true, whatever is noble, whatever is right, whatever is pure,

whatever is lovely, whatever is admirable—if anything
is excellent or praiseworthy—think about such things"
(Philippians 4:8, NIV).

As soon as you awaken or your feet hit the floor
in the morning, say these words out loud: "Today is
going to be a great day." Because your mind is prone
to negativity, it will find
stress in the upcoming day
unless you train and discipline it. When you direct
your thoughts to "Today
is going to be a great day,"
your brain will help you uncover the reasons why it
will be so. You have a choice in where you direct your
attention, even in times of crisis.

> *Don't believe every
> stupid thought you have.*

Learning how to defeat your ANTs and redirect
your mind with positive thoughts will help you over-
come worry, anxiety, and self-defeatism and live your
best possible life.

CHAPTER 3

STAYING POSITIVE

Harnessing the Power of Optimism, Gratitude, and Love

"Thank you" is the best prayer that anyone could say. I say that one a lot. Thank you expresses extreme gratitude, humility, understanding.

ALICE WALKER

I ONCE HEARD THE FOLLOWING STORY: At the turn of the century a shoe company sent a representative to Africa. He wired back, "I'm coming home. No one wears shoes here." Another company sent their representative, who sold thousands of shoes. He wired back to his company, "Business is fantastic. No one has ever heard of shoes here." The two representatives perceived the same situation from markedly different perspectives, and they obtained dramatically different results.

Perception is the way we, as individuals, interpret ourselves and the world around us. Our five senses take in the world, but perception occurs as our brains process the incoming information through our "feeling filters." When our filters feel good, we translate information in a positive way. When our filters are angry or hostile, we perceive the world as negative toward us. Our perceptions of the outside world are based on our inner worlds. When we're feeling tired, for example, we're much more likely to be irritated by a child's behavior that usually doesn't bother us.

Our view of a situation has a greater impact on our lives than the situation itself. Noted psychiatrist Richard Gardner has said that the world is like a Rorschach test, where a person is asked to describe what he or she sees in 10 inkblots that mean absolutely nothing. What we see in the inkblot is based on our inner view of the world; our perceptions bear witness to our state of mind. As we think, so we perceive. Therefore, in reality, we need not seek to change the outside world but rather to change our inner worlds.

To that end, I teach all my patients the *A-B-C* model:

A = the actual event,
B = how we interpret or perceive the event,
C = how we react to the event

Other people or events (*A*) can't make us do anything. It is our interpretation or perception (*B*) that causes our behavior (*C*).

Consider, for instance, the time I yawned during a therapy session with a patient. He asked if I found him boring. I replied that it was important that he asked. I had been up most of the previous night with an emergency and was tired, but I found what he was saying very interesting. My yawning was *A*, his interpretation that I was bored was *B*, and his asking me about it was *C*. I was glad he asked about my yawn because some patients' C would have been to leave the therapy session with a negative feeling. That's why questioning the *B* stuff is so important.

It can make the difference between a meaningful life and death. Think about the two New Testament stories of Judas and Peter, two of Jesus' disciples, betraying Jesus on the night He was arrested (see Matthew 26:69–27:10). Judas accepted money to identify Jesus to the Temple guards, who arrested Him. Later that night, Peter denied he even knew Jesus—three times.

In both cases, the actual event (A) was their betrayal of Jesus. Judas's interpretation of the betrayal (B) was that he had committed an unforgivable sin; Peter's (B) was shame and remorse. Judas's (C) was to return the 30 pieces of silver and hang himself, while Peter asked for and was given forgiveness and later became a central figure in starting the Christian church. Whereas Peter recognized the possibility for change and redemption, Judas saw

If we don't question our perceptions, they can take us places we don't want to go.

only a dead end. The point being, if we don't question our perceptions, they can take us places we don't want to go.

Optimism + Reality = Resilience

Dr. Martin Seligman, PhD, considered the father of positive psychology, developed a concept known as learned helplessness that has had a powerful influence over my career.[1] He found that when dogs, rats, mice, and even cockroaches experienced painful shocks over which they had no control, eventually they would just accept the pain without attempting to escape. Humans, he discovered, do the same thing.

In a series of experiments, his research team randomly divided subjects into three groups: those who were exposed to a loud noise they could stop by pushing a button; those who heard the irritating noise but couldn't turn it off; and a control group who heard nothing at all.

The following day, the subjects faced a new research task that again involved painful sounds. To turn it off, all they had to do was move their hands about 12 inches. The people in the first and third groups figured this out quickly and were able to turn off the noise. But most of the people in the second group did nothing at all. Expecting failure, they didn't even try to escape the irritating noise. They had learned to be helpless.

Yet—and this is where it gets exciting—about

one-third of the people in group two, who had been unable to escape the pain, never became helpless. Why? The answer turned out to be optimism. Dr. Seligman's team discovered that people who do not give up interpret the pain and setbacks as *temporary* as opposed to permanent; *limited* instead of pervasive; and *changeable* instead of out of their control.

Optimists would say things like "It will go away quickly; it's just this one situation, and I can do something about it."

As a result, Dr. Seligman's team came to believe that teaching optimism could help inoculate people against anxiety, depression, and post-traumatic stress disorder (PTSD).

Here are some of his main ideas.

1. *Listen to yourself and others to see how things are explained.* Are the people powerful or victims? Do they have control or no control? Are hardships permanent or temporary? *Pessimists* describe bad things as permanent and pervasive and good things as temporary, while *optimists* describe things in just the reverse: the bad as temporary and the *good* as permanent and pervasive.

2. *Change your language and feelings around the situations you face.* You can stop being a victim, take control wherever possible, and understand that hardships are usually temporary.

3. *Allow mistakes to be learning experiences, rather than a final judgment on your self-worth.* Everyone makes mistakes; it's how you respond to them that determines how quickly you recover. Accepting a mistake and looking for the lesson you can take away from it will help you get over it and move on. (Remember Judas and Peter?)

Let's look at some of the primary characteristics of optimists and pessimists:

PESSIMISTS	OPTIMISTS
Feel helpless	Feel hopeful
See problems as permanent	See problems as temporary
See problems as pervasive	See problems as limited
See no personal control	See personal control or influence
See failure as a statement about self	See failure as a lesson
Have low self-efficacy	Feel self-confident
Focus on problems	Are forward thinking
Tend to be hopeless	Tend to be hopeful
Tend to give up	Tend to stick with difficult things
Are less proactive with health	Are more proactive with health
Hold grudges	Forgive more easily
Focus on worries and negativity	Are less likely to dwell on the negative

PESSIMISTS	OPTIMISTS
Feel more stressed	Feel less stressed
Are more likely to have insomnia	Are more likely to sleep better
See glass as half-empty	See glass as half-full
Are more withholding	Are more altruistic

While these lists focus predominantly on psychological characteristics, research has shown that the way we view and approach life (positively or negatively) can also have a profound impact on our physical health.

A huge study involving more than 97,000 people found that those who were optimistic had significantly lower heart disease than those who were pessimistic.[2] In addition, women who scored highly on "cynical hostility" were also more likely to develop coronary heart disease.

Optimism is also associated with a higher quality of life,[3] a lower incidence of stroke,[4] improved immune system function,[5] better pain tolerance,[6] and longer survival in lung cancer patients.[7]

Yet as we've seen, blind optimism can lead to early death. The Longevity Project from Stanford University found that people who were mindlessly optimistic died the earliest from accidents and preventable illnesses.[8] Being sleep-deprived led to increased optimism and poorer life choices.[9] College students who were too optimistic had more binge-drinking behavior,[10] and compulsive gamblers were often rated as too optimistic.[11]

The bottom line: It is always best to balance optimism with planning for and preventing future trouble. Being optimistic about eating a third bowl of ice cream with caramel sauce will lead to early death, no matter how much you wish it wouldn't!

The Power of Gratitude

One of the early lessons I learned as a psychiatrist was that I could make nearly anyone cry or feel upset by my questions. If I asked people to think about their worst memories—the times they failed, the incidents where they were most embarrassed, or the day they lost someone they loved—within seconds they would feel bad. But the opposite was also true. If I asked them to think about their happiest moments—the times they succeeded or their experiences of falling in love—they generally started to smile.

Dr. Hans Selye, considered one of the pioneers of stress research, wrote, "Nothing erases unpleasant thoughts more effectively than conscious concentration on pleasant ones."[12] That's why if I could bottle gratitude, I would. Gratitude helps direct your attention toward positive feelings and away from negative ones, and the benefits of feeling and expressing gratitude far outweigh almost all the medications I prescribe, without any side effects.

In fact, a wealth of research suggests that a daily practice of gratitude, which can be as simple as writing down several things we're grateful for every day, can improve our emotions, health, relationships, personalities, and careers.

Focusing on gratitude has been found to increase the activity of the parasympathetic nervous system and decrease inflammatory markers;[13] improve depression, stress, and happiness;[14] reduce stress among caregivers;[15] and, among the elderly, significantly decrease state anxiety and depression as well as increase specific memories, life satisfaction, and subjective happiness.[16]

BENEFITS OF GRATITUDE

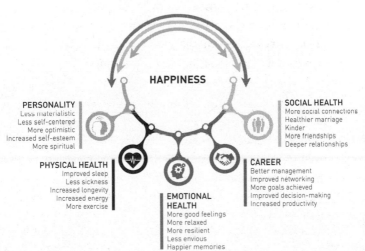

HAPPINESS

PERSONALITY
Less materialistic
Less self-centered
More optimistic
Increased self-esteem
More spiritual

SOCIAL HEALTH
More social connections
Healthier marriage
Kinder
More friendships
Deeper relationships

PHYSICAL HEALTH
Improved sleep
Less sickness
Increased longevity
Increased energy
More exercise

EMOTIONAL HEALTH
More good feelings
More relaxed
More resilient
Less envious
Happier memories

CAREER
Better management
Improved networking
More goals achieved
Improved decision-making
Increased productivity

When you make a habit of bringing your attention to the things you're grateful for, you enhance how your brain works. So, the next time you're feeling stressed or anxious, take a minute to write down three things—big or small—you're grateful for. You might find you have trouble stopping at three.

You can also boost your good feelings if you count your blessings instead of sheep at night. In a study of 221 teenagers, the group that focused on counting their blessings reported increases in gratitude, optimism, and life satisfaction and decreases in negative feelings.[17] At bedtime, write down as many good things in your life as you can think of in three minutes.

While you're at it, get in the habit of writing down the name of one person whom you appreciate and why; then share your feelings with that person with a quick e-mail, text, or call. Do this once a week and try not to repeat anyone for two months.

Or, better yet, write a 300-word essay about someone you are grateful for, such as a teacher, mentor, friend, boss, or coworker. Then, when you have finished, make an appointment with that person and read the essay aloud to him or her. Research has shown that doing this significantly increases life satisfaction scores and happiness and decreases symptoms of depression.[18]

Another exercise that has been shown to quickly increase your level of well-being is called "What Went

Well." Research has shown that people who did this exercise were happier and less depressed at one-month and six-month follow-ups than at the study's outset.[19] Right before bed, write down three things that went well that day; then ask yourself, *Why did this happen?* This simple exercise has been found to help people in stressful jobs develop more positive emotions.[20]

I once treated a very successful businesswoman who made millions of dollars. She was struggling with anxiety and depression, and she felt that she was a failure and that her life was worthless. She repeatedly focused on one incident where a reporter, who as far as I could tell accomplished little in his life except trashing successful people, had harshly criticized her in a magazine article. She played the article over and over in her mind. She had an obsessive pattern in her brain, where she tended to get stuck on negative thoughts and behaviors.

Her first homework assignment was to write out her accomplishments in as much detail as she liked. At her next session she brought eight pages full of accomplishments, including employing 500 people, doing charity work, and maintaining strong relationships. The exercise made her feel great and quickly changed her focus.

Write down the highest and most positive moments of your life. If you can find one moment, odds are you can find two. If you find two, you will likely find four, and so on.

Love—Your Secret Weapon

When Jesus told us to love each other as ourselves, He was giving us good health advice. Research suggests that whenever you feel down, anxious, or angry, it is best to get outside yourself to change your state of mind. In a new study, people who wrote about gratitude activated a part of their brains involved in happiness and altruism.[21]

That said, if you want to feel better, go to the aid of someone who needs help. According to a *New York Times* story, in the 1970s, former First Lady Barbara Bush became so depressed that she sometimes stopped her car on the side of the road for fear that she might deliberately crash the vehicle into a tree or an oncoming car. Mrs. Bush did not seek psychiatric help or medication for her depression, which she blamed on the hormonal changes of menopause and the stress of her husband's job as CIA director. Instead, she said she treated her depression by immersing herself in volunteer work and getting outside herself to help others.[22]

Being loving to strangers—or even to people you know—has the added benefit of making you feel happier, according to two studies. In one study, 86 participants were asked about their life satisfaction and then divided into three groups. The first group was told to do an act of kindness every day for 10 days; the second group was told to do something new every day for 10 days; and the third group was given no instruction. When the 10 days had passed, the groups were retested on life satisfaction. Levels of happiness increased significantly and nearly equally among participants in the groups that had performed acts of kindness or novel activities, while happiness didn't change at all in the group that did neither.[23] Doing something for others for 10 days, especially if you vary the good deeds, is an effective way to make yourself feel better, the study suggests.

Being loving to strangers—or even to people you know—has the added benefit of making you feel happier.

In another study, participants were divided into two groups and asked to recall either the last time they spent either $20 or $100 on themselves or the last time they had spent the same amount on someone else. After completing a scale measuring their levels of happiness, all of the participants were provided with a small sum of money and given the option of spending the money on themselves or on another person. The researchers found that study subjects were happier when they were asked to recall a time when they had purchased something for someone else, no matter the price of the gift. What's more, the happier they felt about being generous in the past, the greater the likelihood that they would spend money on someone besides themselves.[24] As the Bible states, "it is more blessed to give than to receive" (Acts 20:35).

Turn toward Others

Finally, research shows the happiest people are outward facing, focusing more on the people they serve than on themselves.[25]

Even though the prayer attributed to St. Francis of Assisi was likely not written by him, it still provides a research-based guide to happiness. The next time you feel stressed, consider repeating it or any other similar prayer or meditation, such as the Loving-Kindness Meditation.

> **PEACE PRAYER OF ST. FRANCIS**
> *Lord, make me an instrument of your peace:*
> *where there is hatred, let me sow love;*
> *where there is injury, pardon;*
> *where there is doubt, faith;*
> *where there is despair, hope;*
> *where there is darkness, light;*
> *where there is sadness, joy.*
>
> *O divine Master, grant that I may not so much seek*
> *to be consoled as to console,*
> *to be understood as to understand,*
> *to be loved as to love.*

For it is in giving that we receive,
it is in pardoning that we are pardoned,
and it is in dying that we are born to eternal life.
Amen.

By consciously bringing your attention to what you are grateful for—the people who bring you joy and your own successes—you'll see a decrease in worry, anxiety, anger, and negativity and be on your way to feeling better fast.

CHAPTER 4

THE SECRET

Conquering Anxiety for a Lifetime

*The chief function of the body is
to carry the brain around.*

THOMAS EDISON

Up to this point, we have been focusing on techniques and strategies to help you feel better, less anxious, and more emotionally centered "right now." We've discussed breathing techniques and visualization exercises to help you calm yourself down in a crisis; we've taken a long, hard look at the destructive power of automatic negative thoughts (ANTs) and explored practical strategies to combat them; and we've talked about the healing power of love and gratitude.

But as a psychiatrist and brain imaging specialist, I can assure you that the secret to overcoming anxiety both now and for the rest of your life is to work on optimizing the physical functioning of your brain.

The Missing Piece

Physicians have been trying to drug the brain into submission since the 1950s. The outcomes have been poor because doctors too often ignore the necessity of first putting the brain into a healing environment by addressing issues such as sleep, toxins, diet, exercise, and supplementation.

Dr. Thomas Insel, former director of the National Institute of Mental Health, wrote, "The unfortunate reality is that current medications help too few people to get better and very few people to get well."[1] In contrast with antibiotics, which can cure infections, none of the medications for the mind cure anything. They provide only a temporary bandage that comes off when the psychotropic medications are stopped, causing symptoms to recur. In addition, many of these medications are insidious; once you start on them, they change your brain chemistry so you need them in order to feel normal.

Honestly, I, too, undervalued brain health for nearly a decade as a young psychiatrist until our group at Amen Clinics found a practical way to look at the brain. Before we started our brain imaging work in 1991, I had been trained and board-certified as a child and adolescent psychiatrist and general psychiatrist and was busy seeing children, teens, adults, and older adults with a wide variety of issues connected with mental health, including depression, bipolar disorder, autism, violence, marital conflict, school failure, and ADHD.

During that time, I was flying blind and not thinking much about the actual physical functioning of my patients' brains. Researchers at academic centers told us that brain imaging tools were not ready for clinical practice—maybe someday in the future.

I loved being a psychiatrist, but I knew we were missing important puzzle pieces. Psychiatry was, and unfortunately remains, a soft, ambiguous science, with many competing theories about what causes the troubles our patients experience.

During medical school, my psychiatric residency, and my child and adolescent psychiatry fellowship, I was taught that while we really didn't know what caused psychiatric illnesses, they were likely the result of a combination of factors, including:

- **Genetics**—but no one knew exactly which genes were the real troublemakers;
- **Abnormal brain chemistry**—which gave us many medications to try, but they worked only some of the time;
- **Toxic parenting or painful childhood experiences**—but some people thrived even though they'd been raised in abusive environments while others withered;

- **Negative thinking patterns**—but correcting the erroneous thought patterns helped some people and not others.

The lack of neuroimaging led to a "brainless" psychiatry, which kept my profession steeped in outdated theories and perpetuated stigma for our patients. I often wondered why all other medical specialists looked at the organs they treated—cardiologists, for example, scanned the heart, gastroenterologists scoped the gut, and orthopedists imaged bones and joints—while psychiatrists were expected to guess at what was wrong by talking to patients. *And we were dealing with the most complicated organ of all—the human brain!*

Imaging Changed Everything

In 1991, everything changed for me. My lack of respect for the brain vanished almost instantly when I started looking at the brains of my patients with a nuclear medicine study called SPECT (single photon emission computed tomography). Unlike CT or MRI scans, which look at the brain's anatomy or structure, SPECT looks at brain function.

SPECT basically answers a key question about each area of the brain: Is it healthy, underactive, or overactive? Based on what we see, we can stimulate the underactive areas or calm the overactive ones with supplements, medicines, electrical therapies, or other treatments, all of which optimize the brain. We can also help patients ensure that the healthy areas of their brains stay healthy.

Almost immediately after starting to look at scans, I became excited about the possibilities of SPECT to help my patients, my family, and myself. The scans helped me be a better doctor, as I could observe the brain function of my patients. I could see if their brains were healthy, which meant the issues they were facing were more likely to be psychological, social, or spiritual rather than biological in nature. I could see if there was physical trauma from concussions or head injuries, causing trouble to specific areas of the brain, or if there was evidence of toxic exposure from drug or alcohol abuse (addicts rarely admit to how much they are using, but it is hard to stay in denial when looking at a damaged brain) or other toxins, such as mercury, lead, or mold. I also could see if my patients' brains worked too hard, which is associated with anxiety disorders and obsessive-compulsive tendencies.

I was so excited about imaging that I scanned many people in my own family, including my 60-year-old mother, who had one of the healthiest SPECT scans I had seen. Her scan reflected her life. As a mother of seven children and grandmother and great-grandmother of 44, she has always been everyone's best friend. At the time of this writing, she has been married to my father for 68 years, and she is consistently loving, attached, focused, and successful in every way, including being the club golf champion and a top golfer for more than 50 years.

After scanning my mom, I scanned myself, and my results were not so good. I had played football in high school and gotten sick with meningitis as a young soldier, plus I had a lot of bad brain habits, such as not sleeping more than four hours a night, struggling with being overweight, eating junk food, and being chronically stressed at home and at work. Seeing my mom's scan and then my own, I fell in love with my brain and vowed to make it better. Much of my life after that moment has been about making my brain better and teaching others what I learned about how to do it. When my brain was rescanned 20 years later, it was much healthier.

Now, close to 30 years after we started to look at the brain at Amen Clinics, we have built the world's largest database of nearly 160,000 brain SPECT scans on patients from 121 countries. Our work has clearly taught us that unhealthy brain function is associated with a higher incidence of:

- sadness
- anxiety
- fear
- panic
- brain fog

- poor focus
- addictions
- domestic violence
- incarceration
- loneliness
- suicidal behaviors

- violence
- school failure

- divorce
- dementia

By contrast, healthy brain function is correlated with improved:

- happiness
- joy
- energy
- resilience
- focus

- longevity
- relationships
- school performance
- business success
- wealth management
- creativity

Simply put, as your brain becomes healthier, you will experience fewer of the problems on the first list and more of the rewards on the second. And as these positive personal characteristics take hold, you'll experience constructive changes in your attitude, your ability to respond to challenges, and your sense of purpose.

The Most Important Question You Can Ask Yourself

To truly feel and be your best, you need to love and care for the three-pound supercomputer between your ears. Yet very few people really care about their brains, likely because they cannot see them. You can see the wrinkles in your skin, the fat around your belly, the flab on your arms, or the graying hair around your temples. But because very few people ever really look at their brains (via imaging studies), many just don't pay attention to them. As a result, they don't care about them, which is why they tend to develop unhealthy habits like drinking too much alcohol, smoking pot, eating low-quality fast food on the run, and not making sleep a priority.

But once you truly love your brain, everything in your life changes because you have a heightened sense of urgency to care for it. Think about it. If you had a $300,000 Ferrari, would you ever pour sugar or salt into the gas tank? Would you run it until it couldn't go anymore without maintenance? Of course not! Well . . . isn't your brain worth so much more? Of course it is! Your brain needs you to love and care for it, or it will never be able to fully take care of you.

Ask yourself, Is the decision I'm about to make good for my brain or bad for it?

So how can you start loving your brain right here and now? It's actually very simple. *Whenever you come to a decision point in your day, ask yourself, Is the decision I'm about to make good for my brain or bad for it?*

For example, let's say you just had a fight with your spouse. Should you

1. respond in anger and tell him or her exactly what's on your mind?
2. have a donut to calm your nerves?
3. grab an apple and a few nuts, and take a walk to calm down and consider what you can do to make the situation better?

Or what if your stock portfolio went down after a stock market sell-off? Should you

1. stay up all night to figure out your next best move?
2. make sure you get seven hours of sleep so you are well rested and can make good decisions about your stocks the next day?
3. smoke a joint to relax?

One more: Pretend your boss just told you she was unhappy with your performance. Should you

1. skip lunch, put your head down, and work harder?
2. complain to your coworkers about how unreasonable your boss is over a beer and nachos after work?
3. take a walk to clear your head, and when you return, ask your boss for feedback on how you can improve?

It's really pretty straightforward if you think about it, isn't it? The bottom line is this: If you make a habit of asking, *Is this decision good for my brain or bad for it?* at the moment of choice and then make the decision that is in the best interest of the health of your brain, you'll feel better, be less anxious, and be more fully equipped to handle whatever challenges come your way.

Avoid anything that hurts your brain

One of the world's richest men, Warren Buffett, famed business investor and CEO of Berkshire Hathaway, has two rules of investing:

Rule #1: Never lose money
Rule #2: Never forget rule #1

Likewise, here are the most important rules of brain health:

Rule #1: Never lose brain cells
Rule #2: Never forget rule #1

Trust me, losing brain cells is *much* harder to recover from than any financial loss. Just ask anyone who has had a serious brain injury or a stroke.

When I was in medical school, we were taught that people were born with all the brain cells they would ever have, and once those were gone, that was it. While we now know that is not completely true, only certain small areas of the brain make new cells every day. That's why you should do everything you can to avoid losing the brain cells you have.

In my book *Memory Rescue: Supercharge Your Brain, Reverse Memory Loss, and Remember What Matters Most*, I developed the mnemonic BRIGHT MINDS to help you remember the 11 major factors that steal brain cells and lead to cognitive impairment. You can prevent or treat almost all these risk factors, and even the ones that you can't (such as genetic predisposition) can be ameliorated with the right strategies.

Here is a brief summary of the BRIGHT MINDS risk factors. Risks marked with an asterisk (*) are things that might make us *feel* better temporarily but will hurt us in the long run.

B – Blood flow: Circulation is essential to life. It is the conduit for transporting nutrients to, and toxins away from, your cells. Low blood flow shrinks the brain and kills its cells. In fact, low blood flow on brain imaging is the number one predictor of future Alzheimer's disease. What's more, if you have blood flow problems anywhere, you likely have them throughout your body.

Blood Flow Risks That Drain Your Brain

- Excessive caffeine*
- Nicotine*
- Dehydration
- Hypertension
- Too little exercise*

R – Retirement/aging: The risk of brain dysfunction increases with age. When you stop learning or connecting with others, your brain starts dying.

Retirement/Aging Risks That Drain Your Brain

- Loneliness or social isolation
- Being in a job that does not require new learning
- Retirement without new learning endeavors

I – Inflammation: Chronic inflammation is like a low-level fire in your body that destroys your organs. Here's a list of inflammation promoters.

Inflammation Risks That Drain Your Brain

- Leaky gut
- Gum disease
- Low omega-3 fatty acids
- High omega-6 fatty acids
- High C-reactive protein

- Fast and processed food, pro-inflammatory diet*

G – Genetics: Your inheritance matters, but your lifestyle matters more. As we will see, genetic risk is not a death sentence; it should be a wake-up call to get serious about brain health.

Genetic Risks That Drain Your Brain

- Family member with cognitive impairment, dementia, Parkinson's disease, or a mental health issue
- Apolipoprotein E (*APOE*) e4 gene (one or two copies raise your risk for cognitive problems)

H – Head trauma: Your brain is soft, about the consistency of soft butter, and it is housed in a very hard skull with multiple sharp, bony ridges. Head injuries, such as concussions, even mild ones, can kill brain cells and cause significant, lasting cognitive problems.

Head Trauma Risks That Drain Your Brain

- History of one or more head injuries with or without loss of consciousness
- Playing contact sports,* even without a concussion

- Activities that increase the risk of brain trauma, such as texting while driving,* trying to carry too many packages at one time, or going up on any roof (don't, unless it's absolutely safe)

T – Toxins: Toxins are a major cause of brain dysfunction. Your brain is the most metabolically active organ in your body, which makes it more vulnerable to damage from a long list of toxins. Personal care products are particularly dangerous, because what goes on your body goes in and becomes your body.

Toxin Risks That Drain Your Brain

- Nicotine (smoking cigarettes, chewing tobacco, vaping)*
- Drug abuse, including marijuana,* which increases the risk of psychosis in teenagers,[2] decreases motivation and school performance, and decreases overall blood flow to the brain, especially in areas vulnerable to Alzheimer's disease[3]
- Moderate to heavy alcohol use*
- Many legal drugs, such as benzodiazepines, sleeping medications, and chronic pain medications*
- Pesticide exposure in air or food, recently

shown to decrease serotonin and dopamine in the brain[4]
- Environmental toxins, such as mold, carbon monoxide, or air or water pollution
- Personal care products (such as shampoos and deodorants) made with parabens, phthalates, or PEGs*
- Artificial food additives, dyes, and preservatives
- Drinking* or eating* out of plastic containers
- Heavy metals, such as lead or mercury
- General anesthesia (use local or spinal anesthesia whenever possible)
- Handling cash register receipts (plastic coating can get through your skin)

M – **Mental health:** Untreated problems ranging from chronic stress and anxiety to bipolar disorder and addictions are associated with cognitive impairment and early death.

Mental Health Risks That Drain Your Brain

- Chronic stress
- Depression
- Anxiety disorders
- Attention deficit hyperactivity disorder (ADHD)
- Post-traumatic stress disorder (PTSD)
- Bipolar disorder

- Schizophrenia
- Addictions (drugs, alcohol, sex)*
- Gadget addiction*
- Negative thinking

I – Immunity/Infection issues: These are common but often unrecognized causes of brain dysfunction.

Immunity/Infection Risks That Drain Your Brain

- Chronic fatigue syndrome
- Autoimmune diseases, such as rheumatoid arthritis, multiple sclerosis, lupus
- Untreated infections, such as Lyme disease, syphilis, herpes
- Hiking* where you may be bitten by a tick
- Low vitamin D level

N – Neurohormone deficiencies: When your hormone levels are unbalanced, your brain is too.

Neurohormone Deficiencies That Drain Your Brain

- Low or high thyroid
- Low testosterone (males and females)
- Low estrogen and progesterone (females)
- High cortisol levels

- Hormone disruptors, such as BPA, phthalates, parabens, and pesticides
- Protein* from animals raised with hormones or antibiotics that can disrupt your hormones
- Sugar,* which disrupts hormones

D – Diabesity: The term describes a combination of being diabetic or prediabetic and being overweight or obese. The standard American diet is a major cause of diabesity, which contributes to chronically high blood sugar levels. These hurt blood vessels and cause inflammation and hormone disruption as well as the storage of toxins—all of which damage the brain.

Diabesity Risks That Drain Your Brain

- Diabetes or prediabetes
- High fasting blood sugar or HbA1c (hemoglobin A1c)
- Being overweight or obese
- Standard American diet* of processed foods, sugar, unhealthy fats
- Drinking fruit juice* (high in sugar)

S – Sleep issues: All sleep problems are a major cause of brain dysfunction, but especially chronic insomnia and sleep apnea. When you sleep, your brain cleanses itself of debris. Without proper sleep, trash builds up, harming the brain.

Sleep Issues That Drain Your Brain

- Chronic insomnia
- Chronic use of sleep medication*
- Sleep apnea
- Drinking/eating caffeinated drinks or food after 2 p.m.*
- Sleeping in a warm room
- Light or noise at night
- Gadgets* that wake you up
- Irregular sleep schedule
- Anger or being upset before bed

Engage in regular brain-healthy habits

Now that you know what risk factors to avoid, it is critical that you begin developing daily habits to help keep your brain working at an optimum level.

Here are 10 to get you started.

1. **Worry—a little.** According to research, people whose motto is "Don't worry; be happy" die the earliest from accidents or preventable illnesses. Some anxiety is good. Obviously too much is bad, but so is too little. Make yourself less vulnerable to poor decisions. Ultimately, the quality of your decisions determines the health of your brain and body. Be sure to have clear goals, get seven hours of sleep every night, and keep your blood sugar on an even keel by eating protein and

fat at every meal. Low blood sugar levels are associated with poor decisions. And select a healthy peer group. You become like the people with whom you spend time, and being with healthy people who take care of their brains is a good way to keep your own brain healthy.

2. **Eat healthy and exercise.** At least twice a week, engage in regular exercise and healthy sports that require coordination and complex moves (dancing, table tennis, tennis, martial arts without head contact, golf, tai chi, qi gong, yoga). Focus on staying hydrated—drink five to eight glasses of water a day, and replace your morning coffee with decaffeinated green tea. Spice up your food with cayenne pepper or rosemary, and eat up to eight servings of fruits and vegetables a day; there is a linear correlation that this will increase your level of happiness.

3. **Learn something new every day.** Take up a musical instrument; learn some new dance steps, a foreign language, or a new cooking skill. Sign up for a night class at your local community college, or volunteer to teach a class at your local library or community center. Not only will you make a few new friends, but engaging in new activities will help keep your brain sharp and your thoughts more focused.

4. **Watch your head!** Always wear your seat belt when you drive or ride in a vehicle, and wear a helmet whenever you go skiing, biking, rollerblading, etc. Remember, just *one* concussion *triples* the risk of suicide.[5]

5. **Detoxify your body.** Whenever possible, try to buy organic foods and personal products. (Apps such as Think Dirty and Healthy Living can help you scan your personal care products and eliminate as many toxic ingredients as possible.) Limit your alcohol intake to two servings a week, and support the four organs of detoxification:

   Kidneys—drink more water

   Liver—eat detoxifying vegetables such as cabbage, cauliflower, and brussels sprouts

   Gut—eat more fiber

   Skin—work up a sweat with exercise or use a sauna

6. **Practice stress management techniques.** When you wake in the morning, say to yourself, *Today is going to be a great day!* Then write down three things you are grateful for—each and every day. Go for a walk in nature (or at least outdoors),

and whenever you feel mad, sad, nervous, or out of control, write down your negative thoughts. Instead of dwelling on them, meditate on Philippians 4:8 (NIV): "Whatever is true, whatever is noble, whatever is right, whatever is pure, whatever is lovely, whatever is admirable—if anything is excellent or praiseworthy—think about such things."

7. **Build your immunity.** Do an elimination diet for a month to see if you have food allergies (gluten, dairy, nuts, eggs, etc.) that are potentially damaging your immune system. Start incorporating immunity-enhancing foods, such as onions, mushrooms, and garlic into your diet, and add vitamins D, B, C, and E to your daily regimen.

8. **Give your hormones a boost.** As a general rule of thumb, you should have your hormones tested on a regular basis, add fiber to your diet to eliminate unhealthy forms of estrogen, take zinc (to help increase testosterone) and ashwagandha supplements (to reduce cortisol and support the thyroid), and consider hormone replacement when necessary.

9. **Watch your weight.** Maintain a healthy weight, and if you are overweight, develop a plan with your doctor to lose those extra pounds slowly and safely. Start eating a brain-healthy diet consisting

of low-glycemic, high-fiber carbs; leafy greens and brightly colored fruits, berries and vegetables; lean proteins to stabilize blood sugar and cravings; and plenty of healing spices (e.g., basil, black and cayenne pepper, cinnamon, cloves, garlic, ginger, oregano, rosemary, sage, thyme, and turmeric). Know your body mass index (BMI) now and check it monthly, and chew sugar-free gum to boost oxygen and blood flow to your brain.[6]

10. **Get more sleep.** Try to get at least seven hours of deep, uninterrupted sleep per night. You'll find it helps if you cool your home a bit before bedtime, turn off your phone and other electronic gadgets or keep them away from your head at night, darken your bedroom with light-blocking curtains, and take melatonin and magnesium supplements or 5-HTP (if worrying keeps you up) before you go to bed.

Start Small, End Strong

I realize I've given you *a lot* of strategies—not only in this chapter, but throughout the book—but I want you to come away feeling empowered, not overwhelmed. There are so many small daily decisions you can make to improve your brain health and to keep worry and anxiety at bay, and they are all within your reach!

Start with just a few and add others as you go, and before you know it, they'll become fully ingrained habits that you won't even have to think about anymore. As you go through each day, keep that key question in mind: *Is this good for my brain or bad for it?* And always—*always*—choose what's good!

As you conclude this book, I hope you find the courage to love yourself and others enough to make changes in your life, one strategy at a time. Your movement toward brain health will help you conquer anxiety; feel better physically, emotionally, and spiritually; and leave a lasting legacy of love, gratitude, and good health for all those around you.

Getting Professional Help

When is it time to seek professional help?

This is relatively easy to determine. I recommend that people seek professional help when their attitudes, behaviors, feelings, or thoughts interfere with their ability to be successful in the world—whether in their relationships, in their work, or within themselves—and self-help techniques, such as the ones in this book, have not helped them fully alleviate the problem.

What should I do when a loved one is in denial about needing help?

Unfortunately, the stigma associated with "psychiatric illness" prevents many people from getting help. People do not want to be seen as crazy, stupid, or defective, and they often don't seek support until they (or their loved one) can no longer tolerate the pain (on the job, in relationships, or inside themselves).

Here are several suggestions for people who are unaware that they would benefit from help or are unwilling to get the assistance they need:

1. *Try the straightforward approach first* (but with a new brain twist). Clearly tell the person what behaviors concern you. Tell him that the problems may be due to underlying brain patterns that can be tuned up. Explain that help may be available—not to cure a defect but rather to optimize how his brain functions. Tell the loved one that you know he is trying to do his best, but unproductive behavior, thoughts, or feelings may be getting in the way of his success. Emphasize access to help, not the person's defect.

2. *Give the loved one information.* Books, videos, and articles on the subjects you are concerned about can be of tremendous help. Many people come to see me because they read a book or article I wrote, or saw a video I produced. Good information can be very persuasive, especially if it is presented in a positive, life-enhancing way.

3. *Plant seeds.* When someone remains resistant to help, even after you have been straightforward and given her good information, plant seeds

(ideas) about getting help and then water them regularly. Drop an idea, article, or other information about the topic from time to time. Be careful not to go overboard. If you talk too much about getting help, people will become resentful and won't pursue it, just to spite you.

4. *Protect your relationship with the other person.* People are more receptive to those they trust than to those who nag and belittle them. I do not let anyone tell me something bad about myself unless I trust him or her. Work on gaining the person's trust over the long run. It will make her more receptive to your suggestions. Do not make getting help the only thing that you talk about. Make sure you are interested in the person's whole life, not just in potential medical appointments.

5. *Give new hope.* Many people with mental health problems have tried to get help and found that it either didn't work or made them worse. Educate your loved one on new brain technology that helps professionals be more focused and effective in their treatment efforts.

6. *There comes a time when you have to say, "Enough is enough."* If, over time, the other person refuses to get help and his behavior has a negative impact on your life, you may have to separate yourself.

Staying in a toxic relationship is harmful to your health, and it often enables the other person to remain sick. Actually, I have seen that the threat or act of leaving can motivate a loved one to change, whether the problem area is drinking, drug use, or an underlying condition like attention deficit hyperactivity disorder (ADHD) or bipolar disorder. Threatening to leave is not the first tactic I would take, but after time it may be the best approach.

7. *Realize that you cannot force people into treatment* unless they are dangerous to themselves, dangerous to others, or unable to care for themselves. You can do only what you can do. Fortunately, today there is a lot more we can do than even 10 years ago.

How do I find a competent professional?

At Amen Clinics we get many e-mails, social media posts, and calls each week from people all over the world who are looking for competent professionals in their area whose mind-set is similar to mine and who utilize the principles outlined in this book. Because some of these principles are still on the edge of what is new in brain science, such professionals may be hard to locate. Still, finding the right person for evaluation and treatment is critical to the healing process. Choosing the wrong one can make things worse. There are a number of steps you can take to find the best person to assist you:

1. *Get the best person you can find.* Trying to save money up front may cost you a lot in the long run. The right help not only is cost-effective but saves unnecessary pain and suffering. Don't rely on a physician or therapist solely because he or she is on your managed care plan. That person may or may not be a good fit for you, and you shouldn't settle for someone who isn't a good fit. If he or she is on your insurance plan, that's great. Just don't let that be the primary criterion if you can help it.

2. *Use a specialist.* Brain science is expanding at a rapid pace. Specialists keep up with the latest developments in their fields, while generalists (family physicians) have to try to keep up with everything. If I had a heart arrhythmia, I would see a cardiologist rather than a general internist. I want to be treated by someone who has seen hundreds or even thousands of cases like mine.

3. *Get information about referrals from people who are highly knowledgeable about your problem.* Often well-meaning generalists give very bad information. I have known many physicians and teachers

who make light of diet, supplements, and lifestyle interventions. It may help to seek out a functional or integrative medicine doctor, who has specialized training and likely can refer you to other physicians as needed.

4. *Once you get the names of professionals, check their credentials.* State medical boards will have a public record of any legal or ethical trouble.

5. *Set up an interview with the professional to see whether you want to work with him or her.* Generally, you have to pay for a consultation, but it is worth spending time getting to know the people you will rely on for help. If you sense the fit isn't good, keep looking.

6. *Read professionals' writing or go hear them speak.* Many professionals write articles or books or speak at meetings or local groups. If you read their writings or hear them speak, you can often get a feel for the kind of people they are and their ability to help you.

7. *Look for a person who treats you with respect, who listens to your questions, and who responds to your needs.* Look for a relationship that is collaborative and trusting.

I know it is hard to find a professional who meets all these criteria and who also has the right training in brain physiology, but it is possible. Be persistent. The right caregiver is essential to healing.

20 Tiny Habits That Can Help You Feel Better Fast

EACH OF THESE HABITS takes just a few minutes. They are anchored to something you do (or think or feel) so that they are more likely to become automatic. Once you do the behaviors you want, find a way to make yourself feel good about them—draw a happy face, pump your fist, or do whatever feels natural. Emotion helps the brain to remember.

1. Whenever I feel anxious or stressed, I will take three deep belly breaths and imagine a safe haven or place that relaxes me.

2. When I hold my partner's or child's hand, I will think of warmth radiating between us.

3. When I start to feel irritated, I will look at some photos of nature.

4. When I feel upset, I will put on the playlist I developed to feel happy.

5. Before I go to bed, I will pray or do a short Loving-Kindness Meditation.

6. When I approach any meal, I will ask myself if I am getting the nutrients I need to serve my health rather than steal from my health.

7. When I shower in the morning, I will ask myself if I am doing what I can to be a healthy role model for my family.

8. Whenever I am around my friends, I will ask myself if I am modeling behavior that helps their health or makes it worse.

9. When I hold my spouse's hand, I will gently squeeze it and remember that if our habits are healthy, our love life will be better and last longer.

10. When I watch the news, I will be on the lookout for ways to make a meaningful contribution to the health of my community.

11. When my feet hit the floor first thing in the morning, I will say to myself, *Today is going to be a great day.*

12. After an ANT pops up, I will write down my negative thought and ask myself, *Is it true?*

13. After I get home and put away my keys, I will push play on a meditation audio.

14. Before I go to bed, I will count my blessings, listing at least three.

15. After I have a negative thought, I will think of what went well that day.

16. When I face a difficult situation, I will ask myself, *What is there to be glad about in this situation?*

17. After breakfast, I will think of one person I appreciate and reach out and tell him or her in a quick text or note.

18. When I feel anxious, I will practice five diaphragmatic breaths to calm myself.

19. When I start the coffee or tea in the morning, I'll think of three things for which I'm grateful.

20. When I am feeling sad, I will take a walk in nature.

25 Simple and Effective Ways to Combat Worry and Anxiety

1. Start every day with the words "Today is going to be a great day." Your mind makes happen what it visualizes. When you start the day by saying these words, your brain will find the reasons that it will be a great day.

2. Write down three things you are grateful for every day. Researchers found that people who did this significantly increased their sense of happiness in just three weeks.[1]

3. Every day, write down the name of one person you appreciate. Then tell him or her. Appreciation is gratitude expressed outwardly, and it builds positive bridges between people.

4. Limit screen time. Studies report a higher level of depression and obesity with increased time spent with technology.

5. Exercise—it is the fastest way to feel better. Go for a walk or a run.

6. Enjoy some dark chocolate. It can boost blood flow to your brain,[2] help improve your mood, and decrease anxiety. In one study, seniors who ate more of it had a lower incidence of dementia than those who ate less.

7. Listen to music. Just 25 minutes of Mozart or Strauss has been shown to lower blood pressure and stress. Listening to ABBA has also been shown to lower stress hormones—Mamma Mia![3]

8. Choose experiences that give you a sense of awe, such as looking at a sunset or something else beautiful in nature.[4]

9. Drink green tea, which contains L-theanine, an ingredient that helps you feel happier, more relaxed, and more focused.[5]

10. Read an inspiring, powerful novel.[6]

11. Take a walk in nature,[7] which is also associated with reducing worry.[8]

12. Go barefoot outside. It decreases anxiety and depression by 62 percent, according to one study.[9]

13. Listen to a sad song. Really. It was found to increase positive emotion.[10] Listening to lullabies and soothing music also decreases stress and improves sleep.[11]

14. Stop complaining! It rewires your brain to see the negative in way too many places.[12]

15. Spend time with positive people if you want to feel happy.[13] People's moods are contagious. (If you want to feel depressed, hang out with gloomy people.)

16. Do something you love that brings you joy. For me, it is playing table tennis or spending time with my wife, kids, or grandkids.

17. Write down your five happiest experiences, and then imagine reliving them.

18. Engage in activities that make you feel competent.[14]

19. Be patient. People tend to be happier with age, especially if they take care of their brains.[15]

20. Learn to forgive; it can help reduce negative feelings.[16]

21. Help someone else or volunteer; people in one study who did felt happier.[17] And make time for friends.[18]

22. Get intimate with your spouse. Making love with a partner increases overall happiness and decreases stress hormones. In mice, it helps boost the hippocampus.[19]

23. Journal your feelings. It helps to get them out of your head and allows you to gain perspective.[20]

24. Learn to kill the ANTs (automatic negative thoughts). Whenever you feel sad, mad, nervous, or out of control, write down your negative thoughts. Next, ask yourself if they are really true or if they are a bit distorted, making you feel worse. Focusing your mind on positive, rational thoughts will help you feel much better.

25. Practice meditation or prayer. Focusing on Scripture for just 5 to 10 minutes a day is a simple yet powerful way to improve your life. Prayer and meditation have been found to calm stress; improve focus, mood, and memory; help you make better decisions; and reduce feelings of anxiety, depression, and irritability.[21]

Nutraceuticals That Help Alleviate Worry and Anxiety

WHEN I'M TREATING PEOPLE, one question I always ask myself is *What would I prescribe if this were my mother, my wife, or my child?* More and more, after all my years as a psychiatrist, I find myself recommending natural treatments. I am not opposed to medications and I have prescribed them for a long time, but I want you to use all of the tools available, especially if they are effective, less expensive, and have fewer side effects than medications.

My interest in nutraceuticals (supplements with medicine-like health benefits) started after I began using brain SPECT imaging to help understand and treat my patients. One of the early lessons SPECT taught me was that some medications, especially those often prescribed for anxiety, had a negative effect we could see on the scans. Later I learned that some research suggested that a number of these medications increased the risk of dementia and strokes.[1] In medical school I was taught, "First, do no harm. Use the least toxic, most effective treatments." As I looked for alternatives to these treatments to help the children and adults I was serving, I discovered that many natural supplements had strong scientific evidence behind them, with fewer side effects than prescription medications.[1]*

Certain supplements are especially effective at calming and balancing the brain, which can lessen feelings of anxiety. Here are some of my favorites:

Magnesium

Magnesium has a calming effect on neuronal function, is involved in more than 300 biochemical reactions in your body, is vital for your body to make energy, and plays a key role in blood sugar regulation. Low magnesium is associated with seizures, inflammation,

---

* Nutraceuticals do have drawbacks. Although they tend to be less expensive than medications, you may pay more for them because insurance usually doesn't cover their cost. What's more, they are not completely without side effects, and they can interact with medications. Also, some studies have shown that supplements don't always contain what the label claims, which means they may not work or, alternatively, could be harmful. Don't rely on the expertise of a health food store clerk for your supplement information. Instead, research brands online and develop a relationship with one or more, communicating your questions and issues to their technical and quality control staff.

Notwithstanding these issues, the benefits of nutraceuticals (and their relatively low risks compared to medications) make them worth considering, especially if you can get thoughtful, research-based information. I have witnessed targeted nutraceuticals make a positive difference in the lives of my patients, my family, and myself, which is why I take them every day and recommend them.

diabetes, anxiety, and depression.[2] With the standard American diet, 68 percent of Americans do not consume enough magnesium. Some researchers believe that supplementing magnesium can decrease seizure frequency,[3] and others have shown it is helpful for severe stress,[4] migraines, depression, chronic pain, anxiety, and strokes.[5] The mineral is found in green leafy vegetables, such as spinach, kale, and Swiss chard; legumes; nuts; and seeds. In general, foods that contain dietary fiber provide magnesium. The typical adult dose is 50–400 mg a day.

GABA

GABA (gamma-aminobutyric acid) is an amino acid that helps to regulate brain excitability and calms overfiring in the brain. GABA and GABA enhancers, such as the anticonvulsant gabapentin and L-theanine (found in green tea), function to inhibit the excessive firing of neurons, which results in a feeling of calmness and more self-control. Low levels of GABA have been found in many mental health disorders, including anxiety and some forms of depression. Rather than overeating or drinking or using drugs to calm your anxiety, natural ways to boost GABA may help. I often recommend GABA supplements. Researchers report that GABA does not cross the blood brain barrier (a network of blood vessels that protect the brain), but the studies are contradictory,[6] with some showing an increase in alpha brain waves (which indicate a relaxed state).[7] Nonetheless, GABA still has a calming influence on the brain imaging studies we have done. The typical recommended dosage ranges from 100 to 1,500 mg daily for adults and from 50 to 750 mg daily for children. For best effect, GABA should be taken in two or three doses a day.

Saffron

Saffron, one of the world's most expensive spices, is grown mostly in Iran, Greece, Spain, and Italy and traditionally has been consumed to help digest spicy food and soothe irritated stomachs. It also has been used for hundreds of years as a folk medicine for a variety of health problems. In recent years there has been significant research showing that saffron can help boost serotonin and benefit mood,[8] memory,[9] and sexual function;[10] decrease the symptoms of PMS;[11] and, when combined with methadone, help alleviate withdrawal symptoms in patients undergoing treatment for opioid addiction.[12] The recommended adult dosage is 15 mg twice a day.

5-HTP

5-HTP (5-hydroxytryptophan), another amino acid, is a step further along in the serotonin production pathway. It is more widely available than L-tryptophan and more easily taken up in the brain—70 percent versus 3 percent of L-tryptophan. About 5 to

10 times more powerful than L-tryptophan, 5-HTP boosts serotonin levels in the brain and helps to calm ACG hyperactivity (greasing the cingulate, if you will, to improve shifting one's attention). A number of double-blind studies have shown that it is also an effective mood enhancer[13] and appetite suppressor.[14] The recommended adult dose of 5-HTP is 50–300 mg a day. Children should start with a half dose. As with L-tryptophan, it is best to take 5-HTP on an empty stomach to help with absorption. The most common side effect is an upset stomach, which is usually very mild. Start with a low dose and work your way up slowly.

L-theanine

L-theanine is an amino acid uniquely found in green tea. It crosses the blood brain barrier and can increase dopamine. It also increases GABA and serotonin, so it tends to have a balancing effect on the brain. It helps with focus as well as mental and physical stress. The typical dose is 100–200 mg two to three times a day.

In addition to these supplements, I typically recommend the following three nutraceuticals to *all* my patients because they are critical to optimal brain function: a multivitamin/mineral, omega-3 fatty acids, and vitamin D.

Multivitamin/mineral

To feel better fast now and later, you need to give your brain the nutrition it requires. But there is evidence that many people are not getting it: More than 90 percent of Americans do not eat at least five servings of fruits and vegetables a day, the minimum required to get the nutrients you need, according to the Centers for Disease Control and Prevention (CDC).[15] An editorial in the *Journal of the American Medical Association* also asserted that most adults don't get all the vitamins they need through diet alone and recommended a daily vitamin supplement for everyone because it helps prevent chronic illness.[16]

In the past 15 years, there have been more than 25 reports of mental health benefits from multivitamin/mineral formulas consisting of more than 20 minerals and vitamins.[17] In addition, studies show that multivitamin/mineral complexes can help with attentional issues,[18] mood,[19] and even aggression.[20] Two randomized, controlled trials were conducted after the 6.3-magnitude earthquake in February 2011 in Christchurch, New Zealand[21] and the devastating flooding in southern Alberta, Canada, in June 2013.[22] Both trials showed reduced acute stress and anxiety scores in those taking a multivitamin/mineral. In the New Zealand earthquake study, the incidence of post-traumatic stress disorder decreased from 65 percent to 19 percent after one month of treatment, while the control group showed little improvement. These two trials suggest that multivitamin/mineral complexes could be an inexpensive public health intervention for normal populations following natural disasters.

A 2010 study tested the effects of taking a multivitamin versus a placebo on 215 men ages 30 to 55. After a month, the multivitamin group reported improved moods and showed better mental performance, as well as having a greater sense of vigor, less stress, and less mental fatigue after completing mental tasks—essentially making them both happier and smarter.[23] Another placebo-controlled study looked at the effects of multivitamins on 81 healthy children and found that those who took multivitamins performed better on two out of three attention tasks.[24]

Omega-3 Fatty Acids

Omega-3 fatty acids are essential to well-being. Low levels are one of the leading preventable causes of death, according to researchers at the Harvard School of Public Health.[25] Studies have shown that 95 percent of Americans do not get enough dietary omega-3 fatty acids. Low levels of EPA and DHA, two of the most important omega-3s, are associated with:

- Inflammation[26]
- Heart disease[27]
- Depression and bipolar disorder[28]
- Suicidal behavior[29]

- ADHD[30]
- Cognitive impairment and dementia[31]
- Obesity[32]

Unfortunately, most people are low in EPA and DHA unless they are focused on eating fish (which can be high in mercury and other toxins) or they are taking an omega-3 supplement. We tested the omega-3 fatty acid levels of 50 consecutive patients not taking fish oil (the most commonly used source of EPA and DHA) who came into Amen Clinics and found that 49 had suboptimal levels. In another study, our research team correlated the SPECT scans of 166 patients with their EPA and DHA levels and found that those with the lowest levels had lower blood flow, the number one predictor of future brain problems, in the right hippocampus and posterior cingulate (one of the first areas to die in Alzheimer's disease), among other areas.[33] On cognitive testing, we also found low omega-3s correlated with decreased scores in mood. Most adults should take between 1,000 and 2,000 milligrams of high-quality fish oil per day, balanced between EPA and DHA.

Vitamin D: Optimize Your Level

Vitamin D's best-known roles may be in building bones and boosting the immune system, but vitamin D is also an essential vitamin for brain health, mood, and memory. Low levels have been associated with depression, autism, psychosis, Alzheimer's disease, multiple sclerosis, heart disease, diabetes, cancer, and obesity. Seventy percent of the population is low in vitamin D because we are spending more time indoors and using more sunscreen (the vitamin is absorbed through the skin). It is easy to remedy a low level: Get a blood test to check it, and if it is low (below 30 ng/mL), take between 2,000 and 10,000 IU a day. Recheck after two months to make sure your level is in the healthy range.

Bible Verses for When You're Feeling Worried or Anxious

AT ONE POINT OR ANOTHER, all of us experience stress. Though a little stress can be a good thing—it keeps us moving and working—too much can have a negative effect on our brains and can cause worry and anxiety.

In Matthew 11:28-29, Jesus encourages us to let go of our burdens and rest in Him. There is no better way to do that than to spend time praying and quietly meditating on His Word. As you meditate on the following verses, focus on the goal of opening yourself up fully to the calming and restorative presence of God.

Don't worry about anything; instead, pray about everything. Tell God what you need, and thank him for all he has done. Then you will experience God's peace, which exceeds anything we can understand. His peace will guard your hearts and minds as you live in Christ Jesus.

PHILIPPIANS 4:6-7

Don't worry about tomorrow, for tomorrow will bring its own worries. Today's trouble is enough for today.

MATTHEW 6:34

Say to those with fearful hearts,
    "Be strong, and do not fear,
for your God is coming to destroy your
        enemies.
    He is coming to save you."

ISAIAH 35:4

Humble yourselves under the mighty power of God, and at the right time he will lift you up in honor. Give all your worries and cares to God, for he cares about you.

I PETER 5:6-7

Worry weighs a person down;
    an encouraging word cheers a person up.
PROVERBS 12:25

Take my yoke upon you. Let me teach you,
because I am humble and gentle at heart,
and you will find rest for your souls.
MATTHEW 11:29

I know the LORD is always with me.
    I will not be shaken, for he is right beside me.
PSALM 16:8

Can all your worries add a single moment to
your life?
MATTHEW 6:27

I am leaving you with a gift—peace of mind
and heart. And the peace I give is a gift the
world cannot give. So don't be troubled or
afraid.
JOHN 14:27

Don't be afraid, little flock. For it gives your
Father great happiness to give you the Kingdom.
LUKE 12:32

The Lord is my helper,
so I will have no fear.
What can mere people do to me?

HEBREWS 13:6

Give your burdens to the Lord,
and he will take care of you.
He will not permit the godly to slip and fall.

PSALM 55:22

If you remain in me and my words remain
in you, you may ask for anything you want,
and it will be granted!

JOHN 15:7

I tell you, you can pray for anything, and
if you believe that you've received it, it will
be yours.

MARK 11:24

Ask me and I will tell you remarkable secrets
you do not know about things to come.

JEREMIAH 33:3

The Lord hears his people when they call to
him for help.
He rescues them from all their troubles.

PSALM 34:17

Pray like this:

Our Father in heaven,
    may your name be kept holy.
May your Kingdom come soon.
May your will be done on earth,
    as it is in heaven.
Give us today the food we need,
and forgive us our sins,
    as we have forgiven those who sin against us.
And don't let us yield to temptation,
    but rescue us from the evil one.

MATTHEW 6:9-13

We know that God causes everything to
work together for the good of those who love
God and are called according to his purpose.

ROMANS 8:28

In my distress I prayed to the LORD,
    and the LORD answered me and set me free.
The LORD is for me, so I will have no fear.
    What can mere people do to me?

PSALM 118:5-6

Jesus said, "Let's go off by ourselves to a
quiet place and rest awhile."

MARK 6:31

This is my command—be strong and
courageous! Do not be afraid or discouraged.
For the LORD your God is with you wherever
you go.

JOSHUA 1:9

God has not given us a spirit of fear and
timidity, but of power, love, and self-discipline.

2 TIMOTHY 1:7

There is nothing better than to be happy
and enjoy ourselves as long as we can. And
people should eat and drink and enjoy
the fruits of their labor, for these are gifts
from God.

ECCLESIASTES 3:12-13

Notes

INTRODUCTION

1. M. F. Hoyt and M. Talmon, eds., *Capturing the Moment: Single Session Therapy and Walk-In Services* (New York: Crown House Publishing, 2014).

2. A. Akgul et al., "The Beneficial Effect of Hypnosis in Elective Cardiac Surgery: A Preliminary Study," *Thoracic and Cardiovascular Surgeon* 64, no. 7 (2016): 581–88, doi: 10.1055/s-0036-1580623.

3. R. Perkins and G. Scarlett, "The Effectiveness of Single Session Therapy in Child and Adolescent Mental Health. Part 2: An 18-Month Follow-Up Study," *Psychology and Psychotherapy* 81, no. 2 (June 2008): 143–56, doi: 10.1348/14/608308X280995.

4. BJ Fogg, Tiny Habits, http://tinyhabits.com/, accessed April 23, 2018.

5. C. A. Raji et al., "Brain Structure and Obesity," *Human Brain Mapping* 31, no. 3 (March 2010): 353–64, doi: 10.1002/hbm.20870.

6. Fogg, Tiny Habits.

CHAPTER 1: WHEN LIFE FEELS OUT OF CONTROL: QUICK CALMING TECHNIQUES

1. R. Sapolsky, *Why Zebras Don't Get Ulcers*, 3rd ed. (New York: Holt Paperbacks), 2004.

2. H. Jiang et al., "Brain Activity and Functional Connectivity Associated with Hypnosis," *Cerebral Cortex* 27, no. 8 (August 1, 2017): 4083–93, doi: 10.1093/cercor/bhw220.

3. T. Tsitsi et al., "Effectiveness of a Relaxation Intervention (Progressive Muscle Relaxation and Guided Imagery Techniques) to Reduce Anxiety and Improve Mood of Parents of Hospitalized Children with Malignancies: A Randomized Controlled Trial in Republic of Cyprus and Greece," *European Journal of Oncology Nursing* 26 (February 2017): 9–18, doi: 10.1016/j.ejon.2016.10.007.

4. A. Charalambous et al., "Guided Imagery and Progressive Muscle Relaxation as a Cluster of Symptoms Management Intervention in Patients Receiving Chemotherapy: A Randomized Control Trial," *PLoS One* 11, no. 6 (June 24, 2016): e0156911, doi: 10.1371/journal.pone.0156911.

5. P. G. Nascimento Novais et al., "The Effects of Progressive Muscular Relaxation as a Nursing Procedure Used for Those Who Suffer from Stress Due to Multiple Sclerosis," *Revista Latino-Americana de Enfermagem* 24 (September 1, 2016): e2789, doi: 10.1590/1518-8345.1257.2789.

6. L. de Lorent et al., "Auricular Acupuncture versus Progressive Muscle Relaxation in Patients with Anxiety Disorders or Major Depressive Disorder: A Prospective Parallel Group Clinical Trial," *Journal of Acupuncture and Meridian Studies* 9, no. 4 (August 2016): 191–9, doi: 10.1016/j.jams.2016.03.008.

7. B. Meyer et al., "Progressive Muscle Relaxation Reduces Migraine Frequency and Normalizes Amplitudes of Contingent Negative Variation (CNV)," *Journal of Headache and Pain* 17, no. 1 (December 2016): 37, doi: 10.1186/s10194-016-0630-0.

8. A. B. Wallbaum et al., "Progressive Muscle Relaxation and Restricted Environmental Stimulation Therapy for Chronic Tension Headache: A Pilot Study," *International Journal of Psychosomatics* 38, nos. 1–4 (February 1991): 33–39.

9. T. Limsanon and R. Kalayasiri, "Preliminary Effects of Progressive Muscle Relaxation on Cigarette Craving and Withdrawal Symptoms in Experienced Smokers in Acute Cigarette Abstinence: A Randomized Controlled Trial," *Behavior Therapy* 46, no. 2 (November 2014): 166–76, doi: 10.1016/j.beth.2014.10.002.

10. K. Golding et al., "Self-Help Relaxation for Post-Stroke Anxiety: A Randomised, Controlled Pilot Study," *Clinical Rehabilitation* 30, no. 2 (February 2016): 174–80, doi: 10.1177/0269215515575746.

11. S. Brunelli et al., "Efficacy of Progressive Muscle Relaxation, Mental Imagery, and Phantom Exercise Training on Phantom Limb: A Randomized Controlled Trial," *Archives of Physical Medicine and Rehabilitation* 96, no. 2 (February 2015): 181–87, doi: 10.1016/j.apmr .2014.09.035.

12. A. Hassanpour Dehkordi and A. Jalali, "Effect of Progressive Muscle Relaxation on the Fatigue and Quality of Life Among Iranian Aging Persons," *Acta Medica Iranica* 54, no. 7 (July 2016): 430–36.
      M. Shahriari et al., "Effects of Progressive Muscle Relaxation, Guided Imagery and Deep Diaphragmatic Breathing on Quality of Life in Elderly with Breast or Prostate Cancer," *Journal of Education and Health Promotion* 6 (April 19, 2017): 1, doi: 10.4103/jehp .jehp_147_14.

13. Y. K. Yildirim and C. Fadiloglu, "The Effect of Progressive Muscle Relaxation Training on Anxiety Levels and Quality of Life in Dialysis Patients," *EDTNA/ERCA Journal* 32, no. 2 (April–June 2006): 86–88.

14. A. K. Johnson et al., "Hypnotic Relaxation Therapy and Sexual Function in Postmenopausal Women: Results

of a Randomized Clinical Trial," *International Journal of Clinical and Experimental Hypnosis* 64, no. 2 (2016): 213–24, doi: 10.1080/00207144.2016.1131590.

15. X. Ma et al., "The Effect of Diaphragmatic Breathing on Attention, Negative Affect and Stress in Healthy Adults," *Frontiers in Psychology* 8 (June 6, 2017): 874, doi: 10.3389/fpsyg.2017.00874.

    Y. F. Chen et al., "The Effectiveness of Diaphragmatic Breathing Relaxation Training for Reducing Anxiety," *Perspectives in Psychiatric Care* 53, no. 4 (October 2017): 329–36, doi: 10.1111/ppc.12184.

16. R. P. Brown and P. L. Gerbarg, "*Sudarshan Kriya* Yogic Breathing in the Treatment of Stress, Anxiety, and Depression. Part II—Clinical Applications and Guidelines," *Journal of Alternative and Complementary Medicine* 11, no. 4 (August 2005): 711–17.

17. L. C. Chiang et al., "Effect of Relaxation-Breathing Training on Anxiety and Asthma Signs/Symptoms of Children with Moderate-to-Severe Asthma: A Randomized Controlled Trial," *International Journal of Nursing Studies* 46, no. 8 (August 2009): 1061–70, doi: 10.1016/j.ijnurstu.2009.01.013.

18. S. Stavrou et al., "The Effectiveness of a Stress-Management Intervention Program in the Management of Overweight and Obesity in Childhood and Adolescence," *Journal of Molecular Biochemistry* 5, no. 2 (2016): 63–70.

19. T. D. Metikaridis et al., "Effect of a Stress Management Program on Subjects with Neck Pain: A Pilot Randomized Controlled Trial," *Journal of Back and Musculoskeletal Rehabilitation* 30, no. 1 (December 20, 2016): 23–33.

20. J. B. Ferreira et al., "Inspiratory Muscle Training Reduces Blood Pressure and Sympathetic Activity in Hypertensive Patients: A Randomized Controlled Trial," *International Journal of Cardiology* 166, no. 1 (June 5, 2013): 61–67, doi: 10.1016/j.ijcard.2011.09.069.

21. S. E. Stromberg et al., "Diaphragmatic Breathing and Its Effectiveness for the Management of Motion Sickness," *Aerospace Medicine and Human Performance* 86, no. 5 (May 2015): 452–57, doi: 10.3357/AMHP.4152.2015.

22. R. Fried et al., "Effect of Diaphragmatic Respiration with End-Tidal CO_2 Biofeedback on Respiration, EEG, and Seizure Frequency in Idiopathic Epilepsy," *Annals of the New York Academy of Sciences* 602 (February 1990): 67–96.

23. P. R. Mello et al., "Inspiratory Muscle Training Reduces Sympathetic Nervous Activity and Improves Inspiratory Muscle Weakness and Quality of Life in Patients with Chronic Heart Failure: A Clinical Trial," *Journal of Cardiopulmonary Rehabilitation and Prevention* 32, no. 5 (September–October 2012): 255–61, doi: 10.1097/HCR.0b013e31825828da.

24. C. A. Lengacher et al., "Immune Responses to Guided Imagery During Breast Cancer Treatment," *Biological Research for Nursing* 9, no. 3 (January 2008): 205–14, doi:10.1177/1099800407309374.

    C. Maack and P. Nolan, "The Effects of Guided Imagery and Music Therapy on Reported Change in Normal Adults," *Journal of Music Therapy* 36, no. 1 (March 1, 1999): 39–55.

    Y. Y. Tang et al., "Improving Executive Function and Its Neurobiological Mechanisms through a Mindfulness-Based Intervention: Advances within the Field of Developmental Neuroscience," *Child Development Perspectives* 6, no. 4 (December 2012): 361–66, doi: 10.1111/j.1750-8606.2012.00250.x.

25. X. Zeng et al., "The Effect of Loving-Kindness Meditation on Positive Emotions: A Meta-Analytic Review," *Frontiers in Psychology* 6 (November 3, 2015): 1693, doi: 10.3389/fpsyg.2015.01693.

    B. L. Fredrickson et al., "Open Hearts Build Lives: Positive Emotions, Induced through Loving-Kindness

Meditation, Build Consequential Personal Resources," *Journal of Personality and Social Psychology* 95, no. 5 (November 2008): 1045–62, doi: 10.1037/a0013262.

26. J. W. Carson et al., "Loving-Kindness Meditation for Chronic Low Back Pain: Results from a Pilot Trial," *Journal of Holistic Nursing* 23, no. 3 (September 2005): 287–304.

27. M. E. Tonelli and A. B. Wachholtz, "Meditation-Based Treatment Yielding Immediate Relief for Meditation-Naïve Migraineurs," *Pain Management Nursing* 15, no. 1 (March 2014): 36–40, doi: 10.1016/j.pmn.2012.04.002.

28. D. J. Kearney et al., "Loving-Kindness Meditation for Posttraumatic Stress Disorder: A Pilot Study," *Journal of Traumatic Stress* 26, no. 4 (August 2013): 426–34, doi: 10.1002/jts.21832.

29. A. J. Stell and T. Farsides, "Brief Loving-Kindness Meditation Reduces Racial Bias, Mediated by Positive Other-Regarding Emotions," *Motivation and Emotion* 40, no. 1 (February 2016): 140–47, doi: 10.1007/s11031 -015-9514-x.

30. M. K. Leung et al., "Increased Gray Matter Volume in the Right Angular and Posterior Parahippocampal Gyri in Loving-Kindness Meditators," *Social Cognitive and Affective Neuroscience* 8, no. 1 (January 2013): 34–39, doi: 10.1093/scan/nss076.

31. B. E. Kok et al., "How Positive Emotions Build Physical Health: Perceived Positive Social Connections Account for the Upward Spiral between Positive Emotions and Vagal Tone," *Psychological Science* 24, no. 7 (July 1, 2013): 1123–32, doi: 10.1177/0956797612470827.

32. R. J. Zatorre and I. Peretz, eds., *The Biological Foundations of Music* (New York: New York Academy of Sciences, 2001).

33. T. Schäfer et al., "The Psychological Functions of Music Listening," *Frontiers in Psychology* 4 (2013): 511.

34. J. Lieff, "Music Stimulates Emotions Through Specific

Brain Circuits," *Searching for the Mind* (blog), March 2, 2014, http://jonlieffmd.com/blog/music-stimulates -emotions-through-specific-brain-circuits, as cited in B. Goldstein, *The Secret Language of the Heart* (San Antonio, TX: Hierophant Publishing, 2016), 29.

35. C. Grape et al., "Does Singing Promote Well-Being?: An Empirical Study of Professional and Amateur Singers During a Singing Lesson," *Integrative Physiological and Behavioral Science* 38, no. 1 (January–March 2003): 65–74, as cited in Goldstein, *The Secret Language of the Heart*, 29.

36. B. Goldstein, *The Secret Language of the Heart* (San Antonio, TX: Hierophant Publishing, 2016), 31.

37. R. H. Huang and Y. N. Shih, "Effects of Background Music on Concentration of Workers," *Work* 38, no. 4 (2011): 383–87, doi: 10.3233/WOR-2011-1141.

38. M. Hausmann et al., "Music-Induced Changes in Functional Cerebral Asymmetries," *Brain and Cognition* 104 (April 2016): 58–71, doi: 10.1016/j.bandc.2016 .03.001.

39. Y. Ferguson and K. Sheldon, "Trying to Be Happier Really Can Work: Two Experimental Studies," *Journal of Positive Psychology* 8, no. 1 (January 2013): 23–33, doi: 10.1080/17439760.2012.747000.

40. E. Brattico et al., "A Functional MRI Study of Happy and Sad Emotions in Music with and without Lyrics," *Frontiers in Psychology* 2 (December 1, 2011): 308, doi: 10.3389/fpsyg.2011.00308.

41. R. Gillett, "The Best Music to Listen to for Optimal Productivity, According to Science," *Business Insider Australia*, July 25, 2015, https://www.businessinsider.com .au/the-best-music-for-productivity-2015-7.

42. A. G. DeLoach et al., "Tuning the Cognitive Environment: Sound Masking with 'Natural' Sounds in Open-Plan Offices," *Journal of the Acoustical Society of America* 137, no. 4 (April 2015): 2291, doi: 10.1121/1.4920363.

43. L. Lepron, "The Songs Scientifically Proven to Make Us Feel Good," Konbini (website), http://www.konbini.com /us/entertainment/songs-scientifically-proven-make-us -feel-good.

44. Y. H. Li et al., "Massage Therapy for Fibromyalgia: A Systematic Review and Meta-Analysis of Randomized Controlled Trials," *PLoS One* 9, no. 2 (February 20, 2014): e89304, doi: 10.1371/journal.pone.0089304.

45. J. S. Kutner et al., "Massage Therapy vs. Simple Touch to Improve Pain and Mood in Patients with Advanced Cancer: A Randomized Trial," *Annals of Internal Medicine* 149, no. 6 (September 16, 2008): 369–79.

    S. H. Lee et al., "Meta-Analysis of Massage Therapy on Cancer Pain," *Integrative Cancer Therapies* 14, no. 4 (July 2015): 297–304, doi: 10.1177/1534735415572885.

46. S. Babaee et al., "Effectiveness of Massage Therapy on the Mood of Patients after Open-Heart Surgery," *Iranian Journal of Nursing and Midwifery Research* 17, no. 2, supplement 1 (February 2012): S120–S124.

47. S. Khilnani et al., "Massage Therapy Improves Mood and Behavior of Students with Attention-Deficit/Hyperactivity Disorder," *Adolescence* 38, no. 152 (Winter 2003): 623–38.

48. F. Bazarganipour et al., "The Effect of Applying Pressure to the LIV3 and LI4 on the Symptoms of Premenstrual Syndrome: A Randomized Clinical Trial," *Complementary Therapies in Medicine* 31 (April 2017): 65–70, doi: 10.1016/j.ctim.2017.02.003.

49. Z. J. Zhang et al., "The Effectiveness and Safety of Acupuncture Therapy in Depressive Disorders: Systematic Review and Meta-Analysis," *Journal of Affective Disorders* 124, nos. 1–2 (July 2010): 9–21, doi: 10.1016/j.jad.2009 .07.005.

    P. Bosch et al., "The Effect of Acupuncture on Mood and Working Memory in Patients with Depression and Schizophrenia," *Journal of Integrative Medicine* 13, no. 6

(November 2015): 380–90, doi: 10.1016/S2095 -4964(15)60204-7.

50. L. de Lorent et al., "Auricular Acupuncture versus Progressive Muscle Relaxation in Patients with Anxiety Disorders or Major Depressive Disorder: A Prospective Parallel Group Clinical Trial," 191–99, doi: 10.1016/j. jams.2016.03.008.

51. A. Xiang et al., "The Immediate Analgesic Effect of Acupuncture for Pain: A Systematic Review and Meta-Analysis," *Evidence-Based Complementary and Alternative Medicine* 3 (2017): 1–13, doi: 10.1155/2017/3837194.

52. C. W. Janssen et al., "Whole-Body Hyperthermia for the Treatment of Major Depressive Disorder: A Randomized Clinical Trial," *JAMA Psychiatry* 73, no. 8 (August 1, 2016): 789–95, doi: 10.1001/jamapsychiatry.2016.1031.

53. M. Lugavere, "6 Powerful Ways Saunas Can Boost Your Brain," Max Lugavere, https://www.maxlugavere.com /blog/5-incredible-things-that-happen-when-you-sit -in-a-sauna.

54. T. Laukkanen et al., "Sauna Bathing Is Inversely Associated with Dementia and Alzheimer's Disease in Middle-Aged Finnish Men," *Age and Ageing* 46, no. 2 (March 1, 2017): 245–49, doi: 10.1093/ageing/afw212.

55. S. Kasper et al., "Lavender Oil Preparation Silexan Is Effective in Generalized Anxiety Disorder—a Randomized, Double-Blind Comparison to Placebo and Paroxetine," *International Journal of Neuropsychopharmacology* 17, no. 6 (June 2014): 859–69, doi: 10.1017/S1461145714000017.

56. P. H. Koulivand et al., "Lavender and the Nervous System," *Evidence-Based Complementary and Alternative Medicine* 2013 (2013): 681304, doi: 10.1155/2013/681304.

57. S. Kasper et al., "Efficacy of Orally Administered Silexan in Patients with Anxiety-Related Restlessness and Disturbed Sleep—A Randomized, Placebo-Controlled Trial," *European Neuropsychopharmacology* 25, no. 11

(November 2015): 1960–67, doi: 10.1016/j.euroneuro .2015.07.024.

58. P. Sasannejad et al., "Lavender Essential Oil in the Treatment of Migraine Headache: A Placebo-Controlled Clinical Trial," *European Neurology* 67, no. 5 (2012): 288–91, doi: 10.1159/000335249.

59. M. Kheirkhah et al., "Comparing the Effects of Aromatherapy with Rose Oils and Warm Foot Bath on Anxiety in the First Stage of Labor in Nulliparous Women," *Iranian Red Crescent Medical Journal* 16, no. 9 (August 17, 2014): e14455, doi: 10.5812/ircmj.14455.

    T. Hongratanaworakit, "Relaxing Effect of Rose Oil on Humans," *Natural Product Communications* 4, no. 2 (February 2009): 291–96.

60. J. D. Amsterdam et al., "Chamomile (Matricaria recutita) May Provide Antidepressant Activity in Anxious, Depressed Humans: An Exploratory Study," *Alternative Therapies in Health and Medicine* 18, no. 5 (September–October 2012): 44–49.

61. C. Maller et al., "Healthy Nature Healthy People: 'Contact with Nature' as an Upstream Health Promotion Intervention for Populations," *Health Promotion International* 21, no. 1 (March 2006): 45–54.

62. P. Lambrou, "Fun with Fractals? Why Nature Can Be Calming," *Psychology Today* website, September 7, 2012, https://www.psychologytoday.com/blog/codes-joy /201209/fun-fractals.

63. C. J. Beukeboom et al., "Stress-Reducing Effects of Real and Artificial Nature in a Hospital Waiting Room," *Journal of Alternative and Complementary Medicine* 18, no. 4 (April 2012): 329–33, doi: 10.1089/acm.2011 .0488.

64. H. Williams, "9 Ways to Improve Your Mood with Food: Herbs and Spices," AllWomensTalk (website), http:// health.allwomenstalk.com/ways-to-improve-your-mood -with-food/4.

CHAPTER 2: HOW TO FEEL HAPPY AND PRESENT: CONQUERING WORRY AND NEGATIVITY

1. Association for Psychological Science, "Believing the Future Will Be Favorable May Prevent Action," *ScienceDaily*, August 3, 2017, https://www.sciencedaily.com/releases/2017/08/170803145643.htm.

2. K. McSpadden, "You Now Have a Shorter Attention Span Than a Goldfish," *Time*, May 14, 2015, http://time.com/3858309/attention-spans-goldfish.

3. J. Twenge, "What Might Explain the Unhappiness Epidemic?" The Conversation website, January 22, 2018, https://theconversation.com/what-might-explain-the-unhappiness-epidemic-90212.

4. R. F. Baumeister et al., "Bad Is Stronger Than Good," *Review of General Psychology* 5, no. 4 (December 2001): 323–370, doi: 10.1037/1089-2680.5.4.323.

5. J. McCoy, "New Outbrain Study Says Negative Headlines Do Better Than Positive," Business 2 Community website, March 15, 2014, https://www.business2community.com/blogging/new-outbrain-study-says-negative-headlines-better-positive-0810707.

6. R. Williams, "Are We Hardwired to Be Negative or Positive?" ICF website, June 30, 2014, https://coachfederation.org/are-we-hardwired-to-be-negative-or-positive.

7. R. Hanson, "Confronting the Negativity Bias," *Rick Hanson* (blog), accessed March 25, 2018, http://www.rickhanson.net/how-your-brain-makes-you-easily-intimidated.

CHAPTER 3: STAYING POSITIVE: HARNESSING THE POWER OF OPTIMISM, GRATITUDE, AND LOVE

1. M. Seligman, *Flourish: A Visionary New Understanding of Happiness and Well-Being* (New York: Free Press, 2011).

2. S. Wong, "Always Look on the Bright Side of Life," *Guardian*, August 11, 2009, https://www.theguardian.com/science/blog/2009/aug/11/optimism-health-heart-disease.

H. A. Tindle et al., "Optimism, Cynical Hostility, and Incident Coronary Heart Disease and Mortality in the Women's Health Initiative," *Circulation* 120, no. 8 (August 25, 2009): 656–62, doi: 10.1161/CIRCULATIONAHA .108.827642.

R. Hernandez et al., "Optimism and Cardiovascular Health: Multi-Ethnic Study of Atherosclerosis (MESA)," *Health Behavior and Policy Review* 2, no. 1 (January 2015): 62–73, doi: 10.14485/HBPR.2.1.6.

3. Mayo Clinic, "Mayo Clinic Study Finds Optimists Report a Higher Quality Of Life Than Pessimists," *ScienceDaily*, August 13, 2002, https://www.sciencedaily .com/releases/2002/08/020813071621.htm.

C. Conversano et al., "Optimism and Its Impact on Mental and Physical Well-Being," *Clinical Practice and Epidemiology in Mental Health* 6 (2010): 25–29, doi: 10.2174/1745017901006010025.

Harvard Men's Health Watch, "Optimism and Your Health," *Harvard Health Publishing*, May 2008, https:// www.health.harvard.edu/heart-health/optimism-and -your-health.

4. E. S. Kim et al., "Dispositional Optimism Protects Older Adults from Stroke: The Health and Retirement Study," *Stroke* 42, no. 10 (October 2011): 2855–59, doi: 10.1161/STROKEAHA.111.613448.

5. Association for Psychological Science, "Optimism Boosts the Immune System," *ScienceDaily*, March 24, 2010, www.sciencedaily.com/releases/2010/03/100323121757 .htm.

6. B. R. Goodin and H. W. Bulls, "Optimism and the Experience of Pain: Benefits of Seeing the Glass as Half Full," *Current Pain and Headache Reports* 17, no. 5 (May 2013): 329, doi: 10.1007/s11916-013-0329-8.

7. International Association for the Study of Lung Cancer, "Lung Cancer Patients with Optimistic Attitudes Have Longer Survival, Study Finds," *ScienceDaily*, March 8,

2010, www.sciencedaily.com/releases/2010/03
/100303131656.htm.

8. University of California, Riverside, "Keys to Long Life?
   Not What You Might Expect," *ScienceDaily*, March 12,
   2011, https://www.sciencedaily.com/releases/2011/03
   /110311153541.htm.

9. V. Venkatraman et al., "Sleep Deprivation Biases the
   Neural Mechanisms Underlying Economic Preferences,"
   Journal of Neuroscience 31, no. 10 (March 9, 2011):
   3712–18, doi: 10.1523/JNEUROSCI.4407-10.2011.

10. A. J. Dillard et al., "The Dark Side of Optimism:
    Unrealistic Optimism about Problems with Alcohol Predicts
    Subsequent Negative Event Experiences," *Personality and
    Social Psychology Bulletin* 35, no. 11 (November 2009):
    1540–50, doi: 10.1177/0146167209343124.

11. R. Ligneul et al., "Shifted Risk Preferences in Pathological
    Gambling," *Psychological Medicine* 43, no. 5 (May 2013):
    1059–68, doi: 10.1017/S0033291712001900.

12. H. Selye, *The Stress of Life* (New York: McGraw-Hill,
    1978), 418.

13. L. S. Redwine et al., "Pilot Randomized Study of
    a Gratitude Journaling Intervention on Heart Rate
    Variability and Inflammatory Biomarkers in Patients
    with Stage B Heart Failure," *Psychosomatic Medicine* 78,
    no. 6 (July–August 2016): 667–76, doi: 10.1097
    /PSY.0000000000000316.

14. K. O'Leary and S. Dockray, "The Effects of Two Novel
    Gratitude and Mindfulness Interventions on Well-Being,"
    Journal of Alternative and Complementary Medicine 21,
    no. 4 (April 2015): 243–45, doi: 10.1089/acm.2014
    .0119.

15. S. T. Cheng et al., "Improving Mental Health in Health
    Care Practitioners: Randomized Controlled Trial of
    a Gratitude Intervention," *Journal of Consulting and
    Clinical Psychology* 83, no. 1 (February 2015): 177–86,
    doi: 10.1037/a0037895.

16. E. Ramírez et al., "A Program of Positive Intervention in the Elderly: Memories, Gratitude and Forgiveness," *Aging and Mental Health* 18, no. 4 (May 2014): 463–70, doi: 10.1080/13607863.2013.856858.

17. J. J. Froh et al., "Counting Blessings in Early Adolescents: An Experimental Study of Gratitude and Subjective Well-Being," *Journal of School Psychology* 46, no. 2 (April 2008): 213–33, doi: 10.1016/j.jsp.2007.03.005.

18. S. M. Toepfer et al., "Letters of Gratitude: Further Evidence for Author Benefits," *Journal of Happiness Studies* 13, no. 1 (March 2012): 187–201.

19. M. E. Seligman et al., "Positive Psychology Progress: Empirical Validation of Interventions," *American Psychologist* 60, no. 5 (July–August 2005): 410–21, doi: 10.1037/0003-066X.60.5.410.

20. K. Rippstein-Leuenberger et al., "A Qualitative Analysis of the Three Good Things Intervention in Healthcare Workers," *BMJ Open* 7, no. 5 (2017): e015826, doi: 10.1136/bmjopen-2017-015826.

21. C. M. Karns et al., "The Cultivation of Pure Altruism via Gratitude: A Functional MRI Study of Change with Gratitude Practice," *Frontiers in Human Neuroscience* 11 (December 2017): article 599, doi: 10.3389/fnhum.2017.00599.

22. Michael Wines, "In Memoir, Barbara Bush Recalls Private Trials of a Political Life," *New York Times*, September 8, 1994, http://www.nytimes.com/1994/09/08/us/in-memoir-barbara-bush-recalls-private-trials-of-a-political-life.html.

"Barbara Bush Says She Fought Depression in '76," *Washington Post*, May 20, 1990, https://www.washingtonpost.com/archive/politics/1990/05/20/barbara-bush-says-she-fought-depression-in-76/0ac40655-923e-448d-bfcc-aa3ea5cb88c8/?utm_term=.1bb20fdb6707.

23. K. E. Buchanan and A. Bardi, "Acts of Kindness and Acts of Novelty Affect Life Satisfaction," *Journal of Social*

Psychology 150, no. 3 (May–June 2010): 235–37, doi: 10.1080/00224540903365554.

24. L. B. Aknin et al., "Happiness Runs in a Circular Motion: Evidence for a Positive Feedback Loop between Prosocial Spending and Happiness," *Journal of Happiness Studies* 13, no. 2 (April 2012): 347–55, doi: 10.1007 /s10902-011-9267-5.

25. S. Q. Park et al., "A Neural Link between Generosity and Happiness," *Nature Communications* 8 (2017): 159674, doi: 10.1038/ncomms15964.

   S. G. Post, "Altruism, Happiness, and Health: It's Good to Be Good," *International Journal of Behavioral Medicine* 12, no. 2 (2005): 66–77, doi: 10.1207/ s15327558ijbm1202_4.

   L. B. Aknin et al., "Giving Leads to Happiness in Young Children," *PLoS One* 7, no. 6 (2012): e39211, doi: 10.1371/journal.pone.0039211.

CHAPTER 4: THE SECRET: CONQUERING ANXIETY FOR A LIFETIME

1. T. R. Insel, "Disruptive Insights in Psychiatry: Transforming a Clinical Discipline," *Journal of Clinical Investigation* 119, no. 4 (April 1, 2009): 700–705.

2. R. Douglas Fields, "Link between Adolescent Pot Smoking and Psychosis Strengthens," *Scientific American* (website), October 20, 2017, https://www.scientificamerican.com /article/link-between-adolescent-pot-smoking-and -psychosis-strengthens.

3. D. G. Amen et al., "Discriminative Properties of Hippocampal Hypoperfusion in Marijuana Users Compared to Healthy Controls: Implications for Marijuana Administration in Alzheimer's Dementia," *Journal of Alzheimer's Disease* 56, no. 1 (2017): 261–73, doi: 10.3233/JAD-160833.

4. M. A. Martinez et al., "Neurotransmitter Changes in Rat Brain Regions Following Glyphosate Exposure,"

Environmental Research 161 (February 2018): 212–19, doi: 10.1016/j.envres.2017.10.051.

5. J. Cepelewisz, "A Single Concussion May Triple the Long-Term Risk of Suicide," *Scientific American* (website), February 8, 2016, https://www.scientificamerican.com /article/a-single-concussion-may-triple-the-long-term-risk -of-suicide1/?utm_content=bufferb98ff&utm_medium =social&utm_source=linkedin.com&utm_campaign =buffer.

6. A. P. Allen and A. P. Smith, "Effects of Chewing Gum and Time-on-Task on Alertness and Attention," *Nutritional Neuroscience* 15, no. 4 (July 2012): 176–85, doi: 10.1179/1476830512Y.0000000009.

   C. Lee, "How Chewing Gum Can Boost Your Brain Power," DailyMail.com, April 1, 2013, http:// www.dailymail.co.uk/health/article-2302615/How -chewing-gum-boost-brain-power.html.

APPENDIX C: 25 SIMPLE AND EFFECTIVE WAYS TO COMBAT WORRY AND ANXIETY

1. R. A. Emmons and M. E. McCullough, "Counting Blessings versus Burdens: An Experimental Investigation of Gratitude and Subjective Well-Being in Daily Life," *Journal of Personality and Social Psychology* 84, no. 2 (February 2003): 377–89.

2. M. Ingall, "Chocolate Can Do Good Things for Your Heart, Skin and Brain," December 22, 2006, *Health*, posted on CNN website, http://www.cnn.com/2006 /HEALTH/12/20/health.chocolate.

3. Deutches Aertzeblatt International, "The Healing Powers of Music: Mozart and Strauss for Treating Hypertension," June 20, 2016, *ScienceDaily*, https://www.sciencedaily.com /releases/2016/06/160620112512.htm.

4. E. Brodwin, "Psychologists Discover the Simplest Way to Boost Your Mood," *Business Insider*, April 3, 2015, http://www.businessinsider.com/how-to-boost-your -mood-2015-4.

5. K. Kimura et al., "L-Theanine Reduces Psychological and Physiological Stress Responses," *Biological Psychology* 74, no. 1 (January 2007): 39–45, doi: 10.1016/j.biopsycho.2006.06.006.

6. M. Rudd et al., "Awe Expands People's Perception of Time, Alters Decision Making, and Enhances Well-Being," *Psychological Science* 23, no. 10 (October 1, 2012): 1130–36, doi: 10.1177/0956797612438731.

7. Y. Miyazaki et al., "Preventive Medical Effects of Nature Therapy," *Nihon Eiseigaku Zasshi* 66, no. 4 (September 2011): 651–56.

8. G. N. Bratman et al., "Nature Experience Reduces Rumination and Subgenual Prefrontal Cortex Activation," *Proceedings of the National Academy of Sciences of the United States of America* 112, no. 28 (July 14, 2015): 8567–72, doi: 10.1073/pnas.1510459112.

9. S. Slon, "7 Health Benefits of Going Barefoot Outside," MindBodyGreen website, March 29, 2012, http://www.mindbodygreen.com/0-4369/7-Health-Benefits-of-Going-Barefoot-Outside.html.

10. L. Taruffi and S. Koelsch, "The Paradox of Music-Evoked Sadness: An Online Survey," *PLoS ONE* 9, no. 10 (October 20, 2014): e110490, doi: 10.1371/journal.pone.0110490.

11. Y. H. Liu et al., "Effects of Music Listening on Stress, Anxiety, and Sleep Quality for Sleep-Disturbed Pregnant Women," *Women & Health* 56, no. 3 (2016): 296–311, doi: 10.1080/03630242.2015.1088116.

12. T. Bradberry, "How Complaining Rewires Your Brain for Negativity," *HuffPost* (blog), December 26, 2016, http://www.huffingtonpost.com/dr-travis-bradberry/how-complaining-rewires-y_b_13634470.html.

13. "Can You Catch Depression? Being Surrounded by Gloomy People Can Make You Prone to Illness," DailyMail.com, April 19, 2013, http://www.dailymail.co.uk/health/article-2311523/Can-CATCH-depression

-Being-surrounded-gloomy-people-make-prone-illness
-say-scientists.html.

14. R. T. Howell et al., "Momentary Happiness: The Role
of Psychological Need Satisfaction," *Journal of Happiness
Studies* 12, no. 1 (March 2011): 1–15.

15. C. Gregoire, "Older People Are Happier Than You.
Why?" *Huffington Post*, posted on CNN website, April
24, 2015, http://www.cnn.com/2015/04/24/health
/old-people-happy.

16. M. Mela et al., "The Influence of a Learning to Forgive
Programme on Negative Affect among Mentally
Disordered Offenders," *Criminal Behaviour and Mental
Health* 27, no. 2 (April 2017): 162–75, doi: 10.1002
/cbm.1991.

17. L. Bolier et al., "Positive Psychology Interventions: A
Meta Analysis of Randomized Controlled Studies,"
BMC Public Health 13 (February 8, 2013): 119, doi:
10.1186/1471-2458-13-119.

18. P. Bentley, "What Really Makes Us Happy? How
Spending Time with Your Friends Is Better for You Than
Being with Family," DailyMail.com, June 30, 2013,
http://www.dailymail.co.uk/news/article-2351870/What
-really-makes-happy-How-spending-time-friends-better
-family.html.

19. D. G. Blanchflower and A. J. Oswald, "Money, Sex and
Happiness: An Empirical Study," *Scandinavian Journal
of Economics* 106, no. 3 (2004): 393–415, doi: 10.3386
/w10499.

20. M. Purcell, "The Health Benefits of Journaling,"
PsychCentral website, accessed April 30, 2018, http://
psychcentral.com/lib/the-health-benefits-of-journaling.

21. C. A. Lengacher et al., "Immune Responses to Guided
Imagery During Breast Cancer Treatment," *Biological
Research for Nursing* 9, no. 3 (January 2008): 205–14,
doi:10.1177/1099800407309374.

C. Maack and P. Nolan, "The Effects of Guided

Imagery and Music Therapy on Reported Change in Normal Adults," *Journal of Music Therapy* 36, no. 1 (March 1, 1999): 39–55.

Y. Y. Tang et al., "Improving Executive Function and Its Neurobiological Mechanisms through a Mindfulness-Based Intervention: Advances within the Field of Developmental Neuroscience," *Child Development Perspectives* 6, no. 4 (December 2012): 361–66, doi: 10.1111/j.1750-8606.2012.00250.x.

APPENDIX D: NUTRACEUTICALS THAT HELP ALLEVIATE WORRY AND ANXIETY

1. A. Pariente et al., "The Benzodiazepine-Dementia Disorders Link: Current State of Knowledge," *CNS Drugs* 30, no. 1 (January 2016): 1–7, doi: 10.1007/s40263-015 -0305-4.

   H. Taipale et al., "Use of Benzodiazepines and Related Drugs Is Associated with a Risk of Stroke among Persons with Alzheimer's Disease," *International Clinical Psychopharmacology* 32, no. 3 (May 2017): 135–41, doi: 10.1097/YIC.0000000000000161.

2. J. Anjom-Shoae et al., "The Association between Dietary Intake of Magnesium and Psychiatric Disorders among Iranian Adults: A Cross-Sectional Study," *British Journal of Nutrition* 120, no. 6 (September 2018): 693–702.

3. A. W. Yuen and J. Sander, "Can Magnesium Supplementation Reduce Seizures in People with Epilepsy? A Hypothesis," *Epilepsy Research* 100, nos. 1–2 (June 2012): 152–56.

4. Etienne Pouteau et al., "Superiority of Magnesium and Vitamin B6 over Magnesium Alone on Severe Stress in Healthy Adults with Low Magnesemia: A Randomized, Single-Blind Clinical Trial," *PLOS One* 13, no. 12 (December 18, 2018): e0208454.

5. A. E. Kirkland, G. L. Sarlo, and K. F. Holton, "The Role

of Magnesium in Neurological Disorders," *Nutrients* 10, no. 6 (June 6, 2018): e730.

    E. K. Tarleton et al., "Role of Magnesium Supplementation in the Treatment of Depression: A Randomized Clinical Trial," *PLoS One* 12, no. 6 (June 27, 2017): e0180067.

6. Evert Boonstra et al., "Neurotransmitters as Food Supplements: The Effects of GABA on Brain and Behavior," *Frontiers in Psychology* 6 (2015): 1520.

7. A. M. Abdou et al., "Relaxation and Immunity Enhancement Effects of Gamma-aminobutyric Acid (GABA) Administration in Humans," *BioFactors* 26, no. 3 (2006): 201–8.

8. "Saffron," Examine.com, accessed April 16, 2018, https://examine.com/supplements/saffron/.

    A. L. Lopresti and P. D. Drummond, "Saffron (Crocus sativus) for Depression: A Systematic Review of Clinical Studies and Examination of Underlying Antidepressant Mechanisms of Action," *Human Psychopharmacology* 29, no. 6 (November 2014): 517–27, doi: 10.1002/hup.2434.

9. M. Tsolaki et al., "Efficacy and Safety of Crocus Sativus L. in Patients with Mild Cognitive Impairment," *Journal of Alzheimer's Disease* 54, no. 1 (July 27, 2016): 129–33, doi: 10.3233/JAD-160304.

10. L. Kashani et al., "Saffron for Treatment of Fluoxetine-Induced Sexual Dysfunction in Women: Randomized Double-Blind Placebo-Controlled Study," *Human Psychopharmacology* 28, no. 1 (January 2013): 54–60, doi: 10.1002/hup.2282.

11. M. Agha-Hosseini et al., "Crocus sativus L. (Saffron) in the Treatment of Premenstrual Syndrome: A Double-Blind, Randomised and Placebo-Controlled Trial," *BJOG* 115, no. 4 (March 2008): 515–19, doi: 10.1111/j.1471-0528.2007.01652.x.

12. M. N. Shahi et al., "The Impact of Saffron on Symptoms of Withdrawal Syndrome in Patients Undergoing Maintenance Treatment for Opioid Addiction in Sabzevar

Parish in 2017," *Advances in Medicine* 2017 (2017): Article ID 1079132, doi: 10.1155/2017/1079132.

13. P. Jangid et al., "Comparative Study of Efficacy of L-5-Hydroxytryptophan and Fluoxetine in Patients Presenting with First Depressive Episode," *Asian Journal of Psychiatry* 6, no. 1 (February 2013): 29–34, doi: 10.1016/j.ajp.2012 .05.011.

   J. Angst et al., "The Treatment of Depression with L-5-Hydroxytryptophan versus Imipramine. Results of Two Open and One Double-Blind Study," *Archiv fur Psychiatrie und Nervenkrankheiten* 224, no. 2 (October 11, 1977): 175–86.

14. "5-HTP," Examine.com, accessed April 16, 2018, https://examine.com/supplements/5-htp.

15. Y. Steinbuch, "90 Percent of Americans Eat Garbage," *New York Post*, November 17, 2017, https://nypost.com /2017/11/17/90-of-americans-eat-like-garbage/?utm _campaign=iosapp&utm_source=mail_app.

   "Only 1 in 10 Adults Get Enough Fruits or Vegetables," CDC website, November 16, 2017, https://www.cdc.gov /media/releases/2017/p1116-fruit-vegetable-consumption .html.

16. R. H. Fletcher and K. M. Fairfield, "Vitamins for Chronic Disease Prevention in Adults: Clinical Applications," *JAMA* 287, no. 23 (June 19, 2002): 3127–29.

17. C. W. Popper, "Single-Micronutrient and Broad-Spectrum Micronutrient Approaches for Treating Mood Disorders in Youth and Adults," *Child and Adolescent Psychiatric Clinics of North America* 23, no. 3 (July 2014): 591–672, doi: 10.1016/j.chc.2014.04.001.

18. J. J. Rucklidge et al., "Vitamin-Mineral Treatment of Attention-Deficit Hyperactivity Disorder in Adults: Double-Blind Randomised Placebo-Controlled Trial," *British Journal of Psychiatry* 204 (2014): 306–15, doi: 10.1192/bjp.bp.113.132126.

19. J. J. Rucklidge and B. J. Kaplan, "Broad-Spectrum Micronutrient Formulas for the Treatment of Psychiatric

Symptoms: A Systematic Review," *Expert Review of Neurotherapeutics* 13, no. 1 (January 2013): 49–73, doi: 10.1586/ern.12.143.

20. S. J. Schoenthaler and I. D. Bier, "The Effect of Vitamin-Mineral Supplementation on Juvenile Delinquency among American Schoolchildren: A Randomized, Double-Blind Placebo-Controlled Trial," *Journal of Alternative and Complementary Medicine* 6, no. 1 (February 2000): 7–17, doi: 10.1089/act.2000.6.7.

21. J. J. Rucklidge et al., "Shaken but Unstirred? Effects of Micronutrients on Stress and Trauma after an Earthquake: RCT Evidence Comparing Formulas and Doses," *Human Psychopharmacology* 27, no. 5 (September 2012): 440–54, doi: 10.1002/hup.2246.

22. B. J. Kaplan et al., "A Randomised Trial of Nutrient Supplements to Minimise Psychological Stress after a Natural Disaster," *Psychiatry Research* 228, no. 3 (August 30, 2015): 373–79, doi: 10.1016/j.psychres.2015.05.080.

23. D. O. Kennedy et al., "Effects of High-Dose B Vitamin Complex with Vitamin C and Minerals on Subjective Mood and Performance in Healthy Males," *Psychopharmacology* 211, no. 1 (July 2010): 55–68, doi: 10.1007/s00213-010-1870-3.

24. C. Haskell et al., "Cognitive and Mood Effects in Healthy Children during 12 Weeks' Supplementation with Multi-Vitamin/Minerals," *British Journal of Nutrition* 100, no. 5 (November 2008): 1086–96, doi: 10.1017/S0007114508959213.

25. "Smoking, High Blood Pressure and Being Overweight Top Three Preventable Causes of Death in the U.S.," Harvard T. H. Chan School of Public Health website, April 27, 2009, https://www.hsph.harvard.edu/news /press-releases/smoking-high-blood-pressure-overweight -preventable-causes-death-us.

26. T. A. Mori and L. J. Beilin, "Omega-3 Fatty Acids and Inflammation," *Current Atherosclerosis Reports* 6, no. 6 (November 2004): 461–67.

D. Moertl et al., "Dose-Dependent Effects of Omega-3-Polyunsaturated Fatty Acids on Systolic Left Ventricular Function, Endothelial Function, and Markers of Inflammation in Chronic Heart Failure of Nonischemic Origin: A Double-Blind, Placebo-Controlled, 3-Arm Study," *American Heart Journal* 161, no. 5 (May 2011): 915.e1-9, doi: 10.1016/j.ahj.2011.02.011.

J. G. Devassy et al., "Omega-3 Polyunsaturated Fatty Acids and Oxylipins in Neuroinflammation and Management of Alzheimer Disease," *Advances in Nutrition* 7, no. 5 (September 15, 2016): 905–16, doi: 10.3945/an.116.012187.

27. C. von Schacky, "The Omega-3 Index as a Risk Factor for Cardiovascular Diseases," *Prostaglandins and Other Lipid Mediators* 96, nos. 1–4 (November 2011): 94–98, doi: 10.1016/j.prostaglandins.2011.06.008.

S. P. Whelton et al., "Meta-Analysis of Observational Studies on Fish Intake and Coronary Heart Disease," *American Journal of Cardiology* 93, no. 9 (May 1, 2004): 1119–23, doi: 10.1016/j.amjcard.2004.01.038.

28. E. Messamore et al., "Polyunsaturated Fatty Acids and Recurrent Mood Disorders: Phenomenology, Mechanisms, and Clinical Application," *Progress in Lipid Research* 66 (April 2017): 1–13, doi: 10.1016/j.plipres.2017.01.001.

J. Sarris et al., "Omega-3 for Bipolar Disorder: Meta-Analyses of Use in Mania and Bipolar Depression," *Journal of Clinical Psychiatry* 73, no. 1 (January 2012): 81–86, doi: 10.4088/JCP.10r06710.

R. J. Mocking et al., "Meta-Analysis and Meta-Regression of Omega-3 Polyunsaturated Fatty Acid Supplementation for Major Depressive Disorder," *Translational Psychiatry* 6 (March 15, 2016): e756, doi:10.1038/tp.2016.2.

29. J. R. Hibbeln and R. V. Gow, "The Potential for Military Diets to Reduce Depression, Suicide, and Impulsive Aggression: A Review of Current Evidence for Omega-3 and Omega-6 Fatty Acids," *Military Medicine* 179,

supplement 11 (November 2014): 117–28, doi: 10.7205 /MILMED-D-14-00153.

M. Huan et al., "Suicide Attempt and n-3 Fatty Acid Levels in Red Blood Cells: A Case Control Study in China," *Biological Psychiatry* 56, no. 7 (October 1, 2004): 490–96, doi: 10.1016/j.biopsych.2004.06.028.

M. E. Sublette et al., "Omega-3 Polyunsaturated Essential Fatty Acid Status as a Predictor of Future Suicide Risk," *American Journal of Psychiatry* 163, no. 6 (June 2006): 1100–2, doi: 10.1176/ajp.2006.163.6.1100.

M. D. Lewis et al., "Suicide Deaths of Active-Duty US Military and Omega-3 Fatty-Acid Status: A Case-Control Comparison," *Journal of Clinical Psychiatry* 72, no. 12 (December 2011): 1585–90, doi: 10.4088/JCP .11m06879.

30. C. M. Milte et al., "Increased Erythrocyte Eicosapentaenoic Acid and Docosahexaenoic Acid Are Associated with Improved Attention and Behavior in Children with ADHD in a Randomized Controlled Three-Way Crossover Trial," *Journal of Attention Disorders* 19, no. 11 (November 2015): 954–64, doi: 10.1177/1087054713510562.

M. H. Bloch and A. Qawasmi, "Omega-3 Fatty Acid Supplementation for the Treatment of Children with Attention-Deficit/Hyperactivity Disorder Symptomatology: Systematic Review and Meta-Analysis," *Journal of the American Academy of Child and Adolescent Psychiatry* 50, no. 10 (October 2011): 991–1000, doi: 10.1016/j.jaac.2011.06.008.

31. Y. Zhang et al., "Intakes of Fish and Polyunsaturated Fatty Acids and Mild-to-Severe Cognitive Impairment Risks: A Dose-Response Meta-Analysis of 21 Cohort Studies," *American Journal of Clinical Nutrition* 103, no. 2 (February 2016): 330–40, doi: 10.3945/ajcn.115 .124081.

T. A. D'Ascoli et al., "Association between Serum Long-Chain Omega-3 Polyunsaturated Fatty Acids and Cognitive Performance in Elderly Men and Women:

The Kuopio Ischaemic Heart Disease Risk Factor Study," *European Journal of Clinical Nutrition* 70, no. 8 (August 2016): 970–75, doi: 10.1038/ejcn.2016.59.

K. Lukaschek et al., "Cognitive Impairment Is Associated with a Low Omega-3 Index in the Elderly: Results from the KORA-Age Study," *Dementia and Geriatric Cognitive Disorders* 42, nos. 3–4 (2016): 236–45, doi: 10.1159/000448805.

32. C. Couet et al., "Effect of Dietary Fish Oil on Body Fat Mass and Basal Fat Oxidation in Healthy Adults," *International Journal of Obesity and Related Metabolic Disorders* 21, no. 8 (August 1997): 637–43.

J. D. Buckley and P. R. Howe, "Anti-Obesity Effects of Long-Chain Omega-3 Polyunsaturated Fatty Acids," *Obesity Reviews* 10, no. 6 (November 2009): 648–59, doi: 10.1111/j.1467-789X.2009.00584.x.

33. D. G. Amen et al., "Quantitative Erythrocyte Omega-3 EPA Plus DHA Are Related to Higher Regional Cerebral Blood Flow on Brain SPECT," *Journal of Alzheimer's Disease* 58, no. 4 (2017): 1189–99, doi: 10.3233/JAD-170281.

About the Author

The *Washington Post* has called Dr. Daniel G. Amen the most popular psychiatrist in America, and Sharecare, a digital health company designed to help people manage their health in one place, named him the web's most influential expert and advocate on mental health.

Dr. Amen is a physician, double board–certified psychiatrist, 10-time *New York Times* bestselling author, and international speaker. He is the founder of Amen Clinics in Costa Mesa, Los Angeles, and San Francisco, California; Bellevue, Washington; Reston, Virginia; Atlanta; New York; and Chicago. Amen Clinics have one of the highest published success rates treating complex psychiatric issues, and they have built the world's largest database of functional brain scans, totaling about 170,000 scans on patients from 121 countries.

Dr. Amen is the lead researcher on the world's largest brain imaging and rehabilitation study of professional football players. His research has not only demonstrated high levels of brain damage in players, it has also shown the possibility of significant recovery for many with the principles that underlie his work.

Together with Pastor Rick Warren and Mark Hyman, MD, Dr. Amen is also one of the chief architects of Saddleback Church's Daniel Plan, a program to get the world healthy through religious organizations.

Dr. Amen is the author or coauthor of more than 70 professional articles, seven book chapters, and more than 30 books, including the #1 *New York Times* bestsellers *The Daniel Plan* and *Change Your Brain, Change Your Life*; as well as *Magnificent Mind at Any Age*; *Change Your Brain, Change Your Body*; *Use Your Brain to Change Your Age*; *Healing ADD*; *The Brain Warrior's Way*; *The Brain Warrior's Way Cookbook*; *Captain Snout and the Super Power Questions*; *Memory Rescue; Feel Better Fast and Make It Last*; and *The End of Mental Illness*.

Dr. Amen's published scientific articles have appeared in the prestigious journals *Brain Imaging and Behavior*, Nature's *Molecular Psychiatry*, *PLOS ONE*,

Nature's *Translational Psychiatry*, Nature's *Obesity*, the *Journal of Neuropsychiatry and Clinical Neurosciences*, *Minerva Psichiatrica*, *Journal of Neurotrauma*, the *American Journal of Psychiatry*, *Nuclear Medicine Communications*, *Neurological Research*, *Journal of the American Academy of Child & Adolescent Psychiatry*, *Primary Psychiatry*, *Military Medicine*, and *General Hospital Psychiatry*. His research on post-traumatic stress disorder and traumatic brain injury was recognized by *Discover* magazine in its Year in Science issue as one of the "100 Top Stories of 2015."

Dr. Amen has written, produced, and hosted 14 popular shows about the brain on public television. He has appeared in movies, including *After the Last Round* and *The Crash Reel*, and in Emmy Award–winning television shows, such as *The Truth About Drinking* and *The Dr. Oz Show*. He was a consultant on the movie *Concussion*, starring Will Smith. He has also spoken for the National Security Agency (NSA), the National Science Foundation (NSF), Harvard's Learning & the Brain Conference, the Department of the Interior, the National Council of Juvenile and Family Court Judges, and the Supreme Courts of Delaware, Ohio, and Wyoming. Dr. Amen's work has been featured in *Newsweek*, *Time* magazine, the *Huffington Post*, the BBC, the *Guardian*, *Parade* magazine, the *New York Times*, the *New York Times*

Magazine, the *Washington Post*, *Los Angeles Times*, *Men's Health*, and *Cosmopolitan*.

Dr. Amen is married to Tana. He is the father of four children and grandfather to Elias, Emmy, Liam, Louie, and Haven. He is also an avid table tennis player.

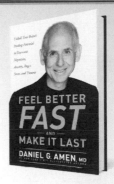
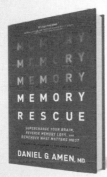
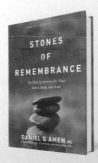